Stephen Damiani has a broad commercial management background across many industry sectors and more recently established his own start-up businesses. He has no college-level medical training and so has had to learn much about genetics and bioinformatics since his son Massimo showed signs of having some rare form of Leukodystrophy. He is very keen to see the promise of precision medicine deliver diagnostic and therapeutic benefits over the next decade. Stephen recently established the Mission Massimo Foundation to promote the prevention, diagnosis and treatment of childhood Leukodystrophies. It aims to accelerate the discovery of novel genetic variations responsible for these debilitating conditions and to translate these findings into clinical treatments.

Sally Damiani has poured her efforts into understanding all she can about Leukodystrophy since first hearing the term in July 2009. Her main focus is keeping Massimo and his twin brothers happy and healthy while she and her husband, Stephen, push for a treatment that will arrest the development of Massimo's disease and even reverse it. In addition to her family, Sally co-founded the Mission Massimo Foundation with Stephen and works in a senior strategy management role with a global healthcare organisation. Prior to this, Sally held strategy, marketing and management consultant roles in Australian and multinational firms.

Leah Kaminsky is an award-winning writer. She is Poetry and Fiction Editor at the *Medical Journal of Australia* and Online Editor at *Hunger Mountain*. She holds an MFA in Creative Writing from Vermont College of Fine Arts. Her novel *The Waiting Room* will be published by Random House Australia in 2015. She is the Damiani family's GP.

CRACKING THE CODE

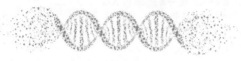

STEPHEN AND SALLY DAMIANI
WITH LEAH KAMINSKY

VINTAGE BOOKS
Australia

Proceeds from the sale of Cracking the Code *will be donated to the Mission Massimo Foundation to promote the prevention, diagnosis and treatment of childhood Leukodystrophies.*

A Vintage book
Published by Random House Australia Pty Ltd
Level 3, 100 Pacific Highway, North Sydney NSW 2060
www.randomhouse.com.au

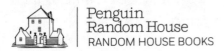

First published by Vintage in 2015

Random House Books is part of the Penguin Random House group of companies whose addresses can be found at global.penguinrandomhouse.com.

National Library of Australia
Cataloguing-in-Publication entry

Kaminsky, Leah, 1959–

Cracking the code / Leah Kaminsky,
Stephen Damiani, Sally Damiani.

ISBN 978 0 85798 466 1 (paperback)

1. Damiani, Stephen – Family. 2. Genetic
disorders in children. 3. Medical genetics.

Other Creators/Contributors: Damiani, Stephen,
author. Damiani, Sally, author.

618.920042

Cover image © Lucie Van Den Berg/Newspix
Cover design by Blue Cork
Typeset in 12/17 pt Sabon by Midland Typesetters, Australia
Printed in Australia by Griffin Press, an accredited ISO AS/NZS 14001:2004
Environmental Management System printer

Random House Australia uses papers that are natural, renewable and recyclable products and made from wood grown in sustainable forests. The logging and manufacturing processes are expected to conform to the environmental regulations of the country of origin.

For the pioneers who embrace the risk of failure as an incredible opportunity for success

CONTENTS

Chapter 1

HOUSTON, WE HAVE A PROBLEM

Sally was six months pregnant when she received an invitation to Victoria's first birthday party.

'When the pretty pink envelope arrived, I ripped it open and saw a tiny, angelic face staring out at me from the card.'

In a year from now, she too would be organising a baby birthday celebration. The whole event was already planned out in her head – down to the colour of the balloons, the style of the cake, the menu and the guest list. The invitations would be pink with white polka dots for a girl; navy, white and red for a boy. What she looked forward to most, though, was the ruckus of kids running around in the yard. She longed for lots of noise in the house.

Fourteen months later, Massimo's first birthday was fast approaching and Sally sat gazing blankly at the screen of her computer, twirling a strand of dark hair around her forefinger; no invitations designed, no matching decorations sourced, no grand first birthday party planned for her son.

'I just couldn't bring myself to do it. I felt a deep sense of unease; as though it wasn't right to celebrate.'

Over the previous few weeks Sally and her husband, Stephen, had begun to notice that Massimo was having difficulty pulling himself up to stand. He had stopped cruising along the furniture, and sometimes when he sat down on the floor to play he toppled over, losing his balance. They were puzzled and concerned. Until then, Massimo had been growing beautifully, reaching all his milestones.

'He rolled when the book said he would roll, started crawling and pulled himself up to stand right on cue. He did all the things kids normally do. He was a really happy baby.'

Suddenly, the developmental milestones they had applauded were vanishing before their eyes. Massimo was born with a minor abnormality at the base of his spine called Spina Bifida Occulta, where the outer part of one or more vertebrae does not fully develop. It's a harmless and not uncommon condition, which most people are unaware they have until it shows up as an incidental finding on an X-ray. But Massimo also had a tethering of his spinal cord at the base of the spine, as well as a single kidney, which was picked up soon after birth during an ultrasound done to check a tiny skin tag in the cleft of his buttocks. It meant he might require an operation to release the increased tension in his spinal cord down the track if there were problems with his development, so he was being carefully monitored by a team at the Royal Children's Hospital in Melbourne.

Sally tried to push her concerns about Massimo's new clumsiness to one side in the days leading up to his first birthday.

'I ordered a huge chocolate cake in the shape of the number one, decorated with blue icing. I busied myself calling our immediate family to come and celebrate with us on the day of his birthday, which fell on a Wednesday.'

She was back working full-time in her senior management role at a large contracting firm.

'Six months after Massimo was born I went back to the office, but worked two days a week from home. I'd always planned to return to work and being part of a fantastic management group, who accommodated all of my needs, made it a lot easier than I realised at the time. After six months of nappies, sleepless nights, bottles and purée, being at work was almost a break.'

When she turned off her computer at the office on the afternoon of Massimo's first birthday, on 22 July 2009, and hurried down the steps of Flagstaff Station to catch the train home, Sally had no idea that she wouldn't be returning to her desk for many months to come.

'My mother was already at our place when I walked in the door. So was Jenna, our next-door neighbour. They had come over to say happy birthday to Massimo, who was standing in his favourite spot, beside the coffee table, playing with Jenna's girls who simply adored him.'

They had been discussing the way Massimo was curling his big toe and turning his feet outwards. Sally, despite her own heightened anxiety that something was not quite right, reassured them, saying she would make sure to ask the physiotherapist to check it out at their visit the following day.

Then she popped Massimo into his highchair to feed him, loaded the *Baby Einstein* DVD and smiled as his face lit up. His favourite cartoon caterpillar crawled across the screen and Massimo squealed in anticipation, flapping his arms and legs in the air.

'It's something he used to do a lot back then, but I never captured it on camera,' Sally says regretfully. 'That excitement on Massimo's face and his yelp of sheer joy have been imprinted on my mind ever since.'

Later that evening, the entire family came over for dinner. Much of the discussion revolved around the changes everyone was noticing in Massimo. After they all sang 'Happy Birthday' and cut the cake, Sally put her exhausted little one-year-old to bed. Walking down towards Massimo's room, they passed her father in the hallway. Soon afterwards, she heard the front door close.

'I assumed he was going outside to smoke a cigar, but when I came back out I found he'd left. All the talk about something being wrong with his grandson had obviously upset him, but rather than show his distress, which we just never did in my family, Dad quietly went home.'

The party finished fairly early and, after they both tidied up the kitchen, Stephen headed off to bed. Sally went in to check on Massimo. She smoothed her hand over his hair, listened to his soft breaths and gently kissed him goodnight. Then she tiptoed quietly into the master bedroom. The house was silent.

Stephen vividly recalls the morning after the celebrations.

'It started like any other day, with the usual organised chaos, except we were all still snacking on the leftovers of Massimo's giant birthday cake.'

Licking some chocolate off his fingers, he downed his third double espresso, threw on his jacket and kissed his son goodbye. He had an important meeting lined up with the sales director of a major men's lifestyle magazine. Business was looking up and Eyre BioBotanics, his newly established organic men's skincare company, had just made significant inroads into Asia and the United States after three years of hard work building the brand from scratch.

Sally stayed home from work to take Massimo to the appointment they had brought forward with Angela Serong, the paediatric physiotherapist who had been seeing Massimo routinely at the hospital since he was six weeks old. The purpose of these regular visits was to monitor Massimo's tethered cord and check he was reaching his developmental milestones. The spinal cord normally hangs loose within the canal, free to move with growth. However, a tethered cord is abnormally attached to fatty tissue at the base of the spine. It causes abnormal stretching of spinal nerves, which can interfere with the transmission of nerve signals to the legs and bladder. Bladder instability was potentially life-threatening, as Massimo only had one kidney. Eventually Massimo would probably need to have his spinal cord operated on, but it was safer to wait until he was older and stronger. In retrospect, the tethered cord was an important sign of things to come, but back in 2009 there was no way of knowing this.

Stephen and Sally were told early on that if they ever noticed a change in the tone of Massimo's lower limbs, such as stiffness in his ankles or toes curling, it could indicate the time was right for intervention. So they requested an earlier appointment, feeling increasingly uneasy about the recent changes.

'It was a dry, cool Thursday afternoon when I bundled Massimo into the car to drive to the physiotherapist,' says Sally. 'Stephen wouldn't normally join us at these sessions, but on 23 July 2009 he decided to come along after his meeting. We saw Angela every three months and our appointments were pretty uneventful; we'd usually spend the thirty minutes marvelling at how well Massimo was doing.'

'Back then, the hospital was a maze of endless corridors,' Stephen recalls. 'Flickering fluorescent globes, timber veneer and frosted glass–panelled walls in extruded aluminium frames, and old service boards with strange plugs from a bygone era plastered with embossed Dymo labels. It had a 1960s institutional feel about it. I remember sitting in the waiting room on the fourth floor while Massimo stood on a tired vinyl floor, playing at an activity table. I stared out the window, down onto a courtyard filled with old site sheds. Appointments usually ran late in the overwhelmed public system and that day was no exception.'

Sally watched Massimo as he played with the blocks at the table. She started to relax, wondering if they had imagined it all. Angela finally appeared, apologising for the delay, and ushered them into her airy room. Sally and Stephen spilled out their concerns and observations regarding Massimo's recent regression in motor skills. The scheduled spinal MRI had been performed a week earlier, and the neuro-surgical follow-up on the Monday hadn't raised any alarms. Massimo crawled across the room and pulled himself up to stand against a couch, just as normal. It was agreed to continue closely monitoring Massimo for another year before proceeding with surgery. Despite this, something didn't seem quite right to Stephen, and in the subsequent days he wrote to three different specialists around the world for second opinions, none of whom noted any abnormality in the MRI other than the tethered cord. Two recommended untethering Massimo's spinal cord on the basis of his toes curling, which they had seen in images Stephen sent via email.

The physiotherapist now took Massimo through a series of tests, checking his reflexes and trying to get him to move from one table to another. His toes were curling sharply and he didn't seem to want to move his feet. Eventually, he lost his balance and toppled over.

'It's unusual that he can't sit any more,' Angela said quietly. 'A kid's milestones shouldn't be going backwards. I don't understand why he's losing skills. I'm going to call his paediatrician.'

Stephen and Sally took Massimo down to McDonald's on the lower ground floor and waited there for further instructions. Sally remembers ordering a café latte for herself and a double espresso for Stephen.

'The hospital coffee was so bad back then that McDonald's coffee tasted good in comparison. Massimo had a little fruit snack bar that I'd brought from home.'

Forty-five minutes later, Massimo was becoming irritable and Stephen needed to get back to work. It seemed no one was going to call them after all. Not wanting to get stuck in afternoon peak-hour traffic, he decided they would head to the car, figuring there was nothing serious to be concerned about. They could make a follow-up appointment for another day, if need be.

Just as they walked out onto Flemington Road, Sally's phone rang. It was Massimo's neurosurgeon, Dr Wirginia Maixner, asking them to meet her straight away in the Emergency Room.

'It was almost a year to the day since our first visit to Emergency, after Massimo's tethered cord was discovered on an ultrasound of his spine and we were sent in for an MRI scan,' Stephen says. 'Among the chaos and confusion of screaming children, anxious parents and the medical staff rushing from one bed to another, the familiar face of Wirginia greeted us and she told us Massimo's spinal MRI from the previous week had now been formally reported. It showed a faint abnormal signal in the thoracic spine, which was initially thought to be an artefact caused by slight movement during the scan. She explained it was possible Massimo had transverse myelitis, generally a dramatic but reversible condition that causes inflammation of the spinal cord. He would need another MRI scan, this time of his brain as well, as an in-patient, to confirm the diagnosis and start immediate treatment.'

They were asked to take a seat and wait.

'We were soon ushered into a bay and met with the on-call neurologist and registrar,' says Stephen. 'They asked a series of seemingly strange questions about increased dribbling and leg stiffness – it was our first introduction to the term "myelin". In hindsight, knowing what we do now, these questions were already suggesting something alarming was going on.'

Massimo had to fast before being given the general anaesthetic required for the MRI scan, so they waited for a bed to become available in the neuroscience ward. Neither Sally nor Stephen felt any sense of danger or urgency. The matter seemed well in hand.

'We were both searching on our phones to gain some understanding of what was happening,' says Stephen. 'Before the smartphone era, using an old BlackBerry wasn't exactly easy or fast. And it was a long few hours trying to keep Massimo entertained. Finally, the anaesthetist, a friendly, tall Englishman with a shaved head, came in and ran us through the paperwork. At around

11 pm we were called down to Imaging; this would be the third time in twelve months I'd entered the MRI room. As soon as Massimo was asleep I was asked to leave. The procedure usually took around forty-five minutes and we would be notified as soon as Massimo was in recovery.'

Stephen and Sally headed down a series of gloomy, long corridors, which eventually led them to the entrance of a waiting room. Stephen remembers the details vividly:

'There were two doors along the entry corridor – one to a toilet and the other to a small meeting room. Beyond that, the space opened out onto a windowless lounge room. A family – a mother and father and two grandparents – sat in the centre of the carpeted room watching the SBS Tour de France coverage on a large plasma TV. They were trying hard to keep the conversation light-hearted while their child was having cardiac surgery. Commentator Phil Liggett's familiar, warm voice filled the room and I occasionally glanced up at the beautiful scenery on the screen. Despite having recently completed a four-hour Tour de France simulation ride at the gym, I wasn't really paying much attention to the race that night.'

A doctor came in wearing theatre scrubs and approached the other family.

'Voila!' he said, in a thick French accent. 'All done. It went just as planned.' He peeled off his surgeon's hat, scrunching it up into a ball. 'I'm going home to have something to eat now and get some sleep. You can relax.'

After more than an hour had passed since Massimo had

gone in, Sally and Stephen began to feel concerned. Lance Armstrong appeared in the starting box and Stephen tried to focus on him to keep calm. He remembers watching every machine-like stroke of Armstrong's as the cyclist completed the Annecy time trial on his signature yellow Livestrong Trek bike.

Stephen and Sally waited almost two hours for the MRI scan to be completed. Finally, at 1.30 am the neuro-surgical registrar, a young Canadian doctor, entered the waiting room and told them he needed to speak with them.

Sally recalls following him into the small meeting room. 'I wondered why he'd taken us in there.'

The doctor didn't offer them a seat, so Stephen and Sally stood next to each other, facing him as he stood with his back to the door.

'It's bad. It has to be bad,' Sally thought. 'This is what they do in the movies when they have tragic news to deliver; they take people into little rooms, speak to them in private, and leave them alone as their worlds fall apart.'

The doctor asked her a lot of questions. Did she breast- or formula-feed? Was she following any special diets during her pregnancy?

'Why was he asking me all this? Did I do something wrong? Had I hurt Massimo in some way? I fought the urge to vomit so that I could concentrate on what he was saying.'

Meanwhile, Stephen pressed the doctor, demanding to know more. There were some concerns with Massimo's MR imaging – the formation of myelin appeared abnormally delayed for his age, which might impact his development or even be fatal.

Stephen was becoming increasingly frustrated with the lack of information.

'Is it serious?' he asked.

'It could be. We don't really know.'

'Is it treatable?'

'Maybe. We can't say right now. Wirginia will explain everything in the morning.'

'I could taste the bile in the back of my throat,' says Sally. 'My first instinct was to run straight to my baby, but I was paralysed by what we were – and weren't – being told. Surely, this wasn't happening?'

The doctor was visibly shaken, but wasn't giving anything away. He clutched his clipboard to his chest and turned to open the door for Stephen and Sally, signalling that the meeting was over.

There were no tears; silence filled the room.

'This was our Apollo 13 moment,' says Stephen, referring to the third NASA moon landing mission back in 1970 that went horribly wrong. 'A cryo tank had just exploded and the master alarm light was flashing. Although uncertain of what was happening, we realised we'd just lost our son.'

As they walked out of the office, Sally was startled out of her stupor by the sound coming from the end of the corridor. It was Massimo screaming.

Chapter 2

LEUKO-WHAT?

On a crisp winter's morning in early January 2003, as snowflakes fell softly onto a Parisian footpath, Stephen and Sally trundled towards the Cluny metro station in the heart of the renowned Latin Quarter. They dragged their luggage down a flight of stairs, on the start of their journey home. When they got off the train at the other end, they emerged into the overcrowded departure hall of Charles de Gaulle Airport. It was a chaotic finale to a carefree honeymoon, during which they had travelled around Europe in a rented Peugeot 206.

'Over those wonderful six weeks we'd made absolutely no plans – no hotel bookings or fixed itinerary,' Stephen says, a smile lighting up his face. 'For once, life wasn't micromanaged and scheduled. Without email or phone calls, we were off the grid. If we liked a certain city we would stay there longer, if we didn't we'd simply move on the same day. At one stage we rejigged our entire trip, setting off in the opposite direction just so I could visit Spider-Point, an Alfa Romeo Spider parts specialist in Germany that was closing the following week for the Christmas break. We drove from Paris to Kappel-Grafenhausen near Freiburg, for almost ten hours straight, just so I could buy parts for my car back home. When we finally arrived, Sally endured another two hours listening to the salesman and me going through a shopping list of parts from camshafts through to suspension.'

By the end of their trip they had covered more than 5000 kilometres, passed through seven countries, stayed in twelve cities, spent Christmas in Munich and New Year's Eve in Berlin. Despite trying their 'just married' status, which had seen them receive many 'honeymoon suite' upgrades across Europe, at check-in for the flight to Singapore it didn't help bump them forward a few rows into Business Class. Instead they were offered the front row of Economy and complimentary One World lounge passes, where they sat together staring out at a snow-covered vista of the outskirts of Paris.

After a couple of hours delay, they finally boarded their flight. As the plane pushed back from the gate, joining the queue for take-off, the fluffy snowflakes were working themselves up into a blizzard. By the time QF18 to Singapore reached the runway, Stephen recalls looking out the cabin window at the snow piled up on the aeroplane's wing.

'I was an avid fan of *Air Crash Investigation*–type TV shows and felt as if I had already seen this episode. The snow wasn't looking quite so beautiful any more.'

The Boeing 747-400 turned onto the runway ready for take-off, but its four Rolls-Royce engines spooled back down to idle. Within thirty seconds, the captain's voice came over the PA, announcing that due to icy conditions the airport had just been closed and they were returning to the gate to await further instructions. In the hope of maintaining the plane's departure slot and minimising what was already likely to be a prolonged delay, the captain had decided that everyone was to remain on board.

The three hundred passengers let out a collective sigh of disappointment. Stephen stretched out, resigning himself to what he knew would be a long wait.

'As the hours rolled past we began to realise both the advantages and disadvantages of our prized seats. Sure, the extra leg room was great, but it was agonising to see those in Business Class being served an endless supply of canapés, washed down with French champagne, while all we got were foil packets of mixed nuts and some bottles of Evian. We watched several films to while away the time, but Austin Powers' *Goldmember* was the one that brought levity to the fact we were grounded on a plane in Paris for eight hours.'

Being seated in the front row of Economy did, however, allow them the luxury of being able to reach forward when the crew weren't looking, and pilfer a few magazines from Business Class to help pass the hours of boredom. Sally flipped through *Vanity Fair*, while Stephen picked up an issue of *Time* magazine from 3 July 2000, which looked as if it had been kicking around the cabin for a couple of years. On the cover was a picture of two men, one balding, the other with glasses and a moustache, wearing lab coats over their shirts and ties. A bold title in yellow type exclaimed: *'Cracking the Code! The inside story of how these bitter rivals mapped our DNA, the historic feat that changes medicine forever.'* The two rival scientists were John Craig Venter and Francis Collins, and the article described their race to sequence the first human genome – mapping over six billion DNA biochemical letters that make up our individual genetic blueprints.

Stephen read the article with interest. It claimed that 'armed with this genetic code, scientists will become privy to the secrets of human health and disease at the very molecular level'. There were promises that this paradigm shift in our understanding of the field of genetics would lead to 'a revolution in diagnosing and treating everything from Alzheimer's to heart disease to cancer, and more. In a matter of decades, the world of medicine will be utterly transformed.' What Stephen was reading about was touted as the glorious start of the genomic era.

At the time it was one of the greatest scientific breakthroughs ever, seen as a project of a similar magnitude to the previous century's achievement of putting a man on the moon. Nowadays, sequencing a genome can cost as little as $1000, with prices dropping all the time. Looking back on it, Stephen muses that reading this article in 2003 and seeing the parallels between the 'human genome race' and the 'space race', planted the seed for what would become, six years later, his own personal journey into the world of genetics.

On the morning of 24 July 2009, the day after little Massimo had the emergency MRI scan, their lives changed dramatically. Sally was seated in the cramped space beside Massimo's cot in the neuroscience ward of the hospital. Stephen had just joined her back at the hospital, after a sleepless night during which he downed half a bottle of Scotch – 'the start of the struggle with alcohol and depression', as he recalls it.

'There wasn't a great deal Sally and I said to one another the night before. It had been a long day and both the volume and density of information we were trying to process during those tense hours had been overwhelming. I don't think we really knew what to say anyway, because we honestly didn't know where to start. There were so many unknowns, it was impossible to break down the situation into manageable pieces, isolate the problem and come up with a solution. We had agreed I would go home to sleep, as we had a corridor full of products ready to be shipped out to the United States and South Korea before the end of the week. I'd try to get everything prepared overnight because Massimo needed 100 per cent of our attention in the next few days. I was also desperate to get home and trawl the internet to learn more about his illness.'

Stephen remembers making his way down from the

ward at 1.45 am. The hospital corridors were deserted, a far cry from the hustle and bustle during the day.

'It was a ghost town. All I could hear was the humming of the fluorescent lights. Normally my mind is racing with a dozen parallel threads of thought, but on this occasion it had simply shut down. I walked out of the hospital into the cold, breathing in the crisp winter air, longing for a cigarette even though I hadn't smoked in years. I made my way down the long driveway outside of Emergency to where we had left the car fourteen hours earlier. It was foggy that evening; eerie halos surrounded the lights in the car park. We lived 10 kilometres from the hospital and at that time of night it took me only twenty minutes to drive home, but it seemed like one of the longest drives of my life.'

Back at home, Stephen stayed up most of the night searching for clues to his son's possible diagnosis. Within the first few minutes of opening his laptop, what he was reading terrified him. He sent an email to friends at 4.38 am, letting them know about the events of the previous twelve hours and preparing them for potential grim news.

'I must have blacked out after that. I woke up around 6 am with a half-empty bottle of Scotch on one side of the desk, and my screen displaying a wide range of MRI scans of children's brains.'

Back in the ward the following morning, Stephen and Sally waited for further news. 'I am handing Massimo's case over to the neurology team for further investigations,' Massimo's neurosurgeon, Dr Wirginia Maixner, told Sally and Stephen during rounds at 7 am. She looked surprisingly fresh, having not left the ward until after 10 pm the night before.

Neither Sally nor Stephen had really thought to ask about the difference between a neurosurgeon and a neurologist until that moment. In fact, they were so exhausted from being up all night, distressed by the thought their son might be dying, that they didn't really understand what was going on.

'Will Massimo ever be able to walk?' asked Sally. 'What will happen next?'

'The neurologists will take it from here,' Dr Maixner reassured them. 'They are far better placed to manage his condition. We do the cutting, but they look after all the wiring of the brain and nervous system. You will be in good hands.'

She quietly moved on to the next patient, followed solemnly by her team.

'At the time, I did not pick up on the subtlety of her message,' Sally says. 'Massimo would no longer be her patient. It was only later that I realised she was telling us she couldn't fix him with an operation.'

Not long afterwards, a softly spoken man wearing a dark blue shirt and brown R.M. Williams trousers and boots walked into the neuroscience ward and headed straight over to the Damiani family. Introducing himself as Dr Rick Leventer, one of the hospital's paediatric neurologists, he squatted down and smiled at their little boy.

'Ciao, Massimo.' He drew the curtains around them.

'As soon as he did that,' Stephen recalls, 'I knew that the news wasn't going to be good. This is what happens when they tell you something terrible.'

Stephen fixed his gaze on the doctor's Frédérique Constant watch, which was fastened with a brown leather wristband. 'I'm terrible with names, but I always remember people by the watch they are wearing.' His mother, Hilda, worked as a computer programmer for the Swatch Group when Stephen was a kid, so he grew up around watches.

'We pounced on the neurologist immediately.' Sally's voice becomes tremulous as the memory surfaces. 'We fired a round of burning questions that had filled our brains since 1.30 that morning – from the moment we were told by the registrar something was wrong with Massimo's MRI scan.'

Dr Leventer listened carefully to Stephen and Sally's questions, politely explaining that the half-dozen or so theories they had already developed, overnight, were all entirely wrong.

'Have you actually seen the MRI scan yet?' he asked.

When they told him they hadn't, he went off to get a printout from the nurses' station. He brought back a copy of Massimo's brain images and pointed to two pale areas on both sides of their son's brain. A new language of complex medical terms entered their vernacular then – *myelin, white matter, T1, T2, hypo-intense, hyper-intense signals* – but the most frightening word they were to hear was Leukodystrophy. Dr Leventer used analogies of electrical wiring to describe the condition, where myelin, the insulation surrounding the nerves in Massimo's brain, was missing or breaking down. This in turn meant signals couldn't travel down the nerve pathways.

It didn't take long before Dr Leventer began repeating the same litany of questions they had been asked the night before: Did Sally follow any unusual diets when she was pregnant? Were Stephen and Sally in any way related? Was there a family history of childhood illness?

'No,' Sally said, wanting to shout at him. No, no, NO! Why on earth did the doctors keep asking all these things? This was the first time anything like this had ever happened to any child in their family, or among their friends.

The neurologist, whom they would soon come to know on a first-name basis, said they would need to send blood work to Adelaide, the results of which might take several weeks to come back. He also wanted to run more tests while they were in the hospital, the first being to look at the optic nerves at the back of Massimo's eyes. At no stage did either Sally or Stephen think they wouldn't have an answer within hours or, at worst, days.

'As they led us out of the ward for an eye examination,' says Sally, 'we passed the beds of several other children, some with their heads bandaged after brain surgery, others who weren't able to move their limbs. I glanced down at the nurses' desk and saw Massimo's pathology request form.'

The strange word Rick had thrown at them suddenly leapt from the page and glared at her. 'Leukodystrophy'.

Chapter 3

INFORMATION OVERLOAD

Seated side by side on a blue vinyl bench in the eye clinic, Sally felt as though they had travelled back in time.

'The room looked tired; as if it had been forgotten by the decorators for decades.'

Massimo was fast asleep in his favourite position, snuggled into Stephen's left shoulder as if soothed by his father's heartbeat. It was close to noon, but no one else had arrived at the clinic yet, so while they waited Sally searched for the word 'Leukodystrophy' on her BlackBerry. Nothing could have prepared her for what she was about to read: 'Progressive neurological condition with loss of skills. Cannot walk or talk, unable to eat, gradual deafness and blindness. Prognosis for infant-onset type particularly poor. Life expectancy typically two to five years.'

As other families gradually began arriving, a young doctor in light-blue scrubs rushed around the now chaotic room, seeing one screaming child after another. Sally kept reading, horrified by the list of dreadful illnesses her son could have – Canavan Disease, Metachromatic Leukodystrophy, Adrenoleukodystrophy, Krabbe Disease, Vanishing White Matter Disease – each one sounded more sinister than the last.

'I tried to figure out which disorder would be the best diagnosis for Massimo; an illness that could actually be treated. I read the information over and over.'

As Sally began to take in the facts, tears streamed down her face. All of these diseases were fatal, each one typically ending in a premature death. Stephen asked her to read the information to him. Her body started shaking as she mouthed the words on her screen.

'Reading it out loud didn't make it any more believable. I was thinking this couldn't be happening to us, to our precious baby boy, to the child that Stephen and I had always dreamed of having.'

After waiting for almost an hour at the clinic, Massimo finally had some drops placed in his eyes. It would take another forty minutes for his pupils to dilate enough for the ophthalmologist to examine him. Massimo's turn eventually came and he screeched so much that it took both Stephen and Sally to hold him down.

'I think I'm seeing a cherry red spot,' the doctor said finally, placing his instruments back onto the table.

Sally and Stephen both tried to calm Massimo down and

when they looked up, the doctor was gone, abruptly running off to surgery without giving them any kind of explanation.

'What the hell is a cherry red spot?' Stephen asked Sally.

She quickly looked it up. Google told them it was a finding in the macula region of the eye that is present in a number of Leukodystrophies.

'We were sent straight back up to the ward, with Massimo screaming hysterically,' says Stephen. 'We were having trouble piecing together and processing the fragments of information flooding in at such an alarming rate, but there was still more to come.'

They were told that the next procedure scheduled was a lumbar puncture, in which a sample of fluid that bathes the spinal cord is extracted with a needle and sent for analysis. Massimo was quickly ushered away into a separate treatment room.

'You won't be able to come in,' the registrar said, standing between them and their baby. 'It's far too distressing for parents to watch.'

They waited outside, leaning up against the whitewashed wall.

'I caught a glimpse of my tiny son being curled up into a ball, held down by a nurse,' Stephen recalls. 'Just before the door was closed, I saw the doctor pick up a large needle. Then a blood-curdling scream penetrated the corridor, like nothing I'd ever heard from Massimo before.'

The nurse emerged after fifteen minutes, carrying their little boy. He collapsed into Sally's arms, completely exhausted from the most horrific twenty-four hours of his short life. He was discharged that evening and they drove home, with Sally in the back seat of the car, unable to leave Massimo's side.

The following morning was a Saturday, and Sally woke at 8 am from what felt like the longest, deepest sleep she had ever had. She rolled onto her back, dozing a little more.

'I could hear Massimo in his room down the hall, chortling in his cot. I smiled as I lay in bed for another minute, listening to the sweet sounds travelling down the hallway. But his happy babbling soon became muffled in my mind, as I remembered a horrid nightmare I'd had the night before.'

It took Sally a few moments to fully wake up. She opened her eyes and stared at the ceiling rose, suddenly realising it wasn't all a dream. It had really happened.

'My gorgeous, singing baby was going to die.'

That morning Stephen downed coffee after coffee, his eyes glued to his computer screen. He was trying hard to work out what they were dealing with, based on a few words from the doctors, a complex hospital discharge summary and two MRI scan reports.

'Those discharge documents may as well have been written in Swahili.'

Together, he and Sally scoured the internet to find out as much as they could about Leukodystrophies, the umbrella term for a group of rare inherited or genetic disorders. Myelin, the fatty, protective coating over nerve fibres in the brain and spine, otherwise known as *white matter*, does not develop properly in these conditions. They learned that the word Leukodystrophy is derived from the Greek word *leuko*, meaning white, *dys*, meaning lack of, and *trophy*, meaning growth. The loss of myelin impairs the ability to transmit signals from within the brain, as well as to the body, and that was why Massimo started to lose skills.

'We read that there were roughly forty known types of Leukodystrophy,' says Sally. 'However, more than half of Leukodystrophy cases remained genetically unclassified – that is, doctors can diagnose the condition with the general term of Leukodystrophy using MR imaging and pathology tests, but do not know the exact genetic cause. At the time, we pushed this piece of information to the side; we were yet to receive test results so at that stage we were still confident of a diagnosis.'

The 'cherry red spot' that the eye doctor had told them about is generally seen in the more aggressive infant-onset forms of the disease, eventually robbing affected children of all their senses. The prognosis with these types of Leukodystrophy is particularly poor.

'Dr Google was in overdrive and what we were reading was terrifying,' says Stephen.

They were shocked to learn that there was no available treatment and certainly no cure in sight. Any intervention was purely supportive, aimed at minimising pain and discomfort.

'You couldn't dream of a more horrific death. Sally and I realised we were going to lose our son in a matter of months or, at very best, a few years. He would become both deaf and blind, and eventually lose the ability to move or even eat.'

Stephen, always the one to spring into action, insisted they needed to call all their friends, but Sally was dreading this, wondering how she was going to break the news.

'What do you say to someone? *Hi, how are you? Yes, hasn't it been cold lately? Oh, and by the way, Massimo is going to die.* It took a few hours before I could bring myself to dial any numbers. I called one of my closest girl-friends first. We skipped over the usual pleasantries as soon as she heard my trembling voice. When I finally managed to tell her the news, she went stone silent. After a minute she told me she had to go, and quickly hung up the phone. She called back a little later, explaining that she had been so shocked by the news, she'd had to run straight to the bathroom to vomit.'

This same friend turned up the next morning with food and her daughter, Victoria. She sat opposite Sally and Massimo on the floor in the living room.

'We both clutched our kids tightly,' says Sally. 'I remember thinking about how many more times I would be able to do this; I guess she was probably busy giving thanks for the health of her own daughter, the angelic Victoria.'

Only fourteen months had passed since Victoria's first birthday party, when Sally had looked down at her pregnant belly, dreaming of the perfect baby she was going to have. Now she had to come to terms with the reality of the terminally ill child she held in her arms.

That weekend the phone didn't stop ringing and a procession of visitors paraded through the Damiani family's home in the leafy Melbourne suburb of Elsternwick. Neither Sally nor Stephen slept for more than twenty minutes at a time, living on cups of coffee by day and glasses of red wine at night.

'We felt we had aged ten years during those two days in the hospital,' says Stephen. 'Although Massimo seemed glad to be home, surrounded by his friends and family, he definitely knew something was wrong. And I could tell he was scared.'

Sally's brother, John, came over on the Saturday night. After Stephen told him his nephew had a neurodegenerative condition that would eventually rob him of all his senses, John innocently asked, 'And then what happens?'

'I remember downing the remainder of a glass of red wine before welling up and saying, "Then he dies."'

'Our friends were well-meaning,' says Sally, 'but the next day everything felt very different. One of my close friends arrived on our doorstep, arms overflowing with food. Her husband had dropped her off, but waited in the car. I found out later that he couldn't bring himself to come in; it was all too much for him. I didn't give it a second thought at the time, but there were others who never visited us again once they learned of Massimo's prognosis.'

Another friend turned up carrying a walker, a present she had bought a week earlier in anticipation of Massimo's first birthday.

'I realised what it was immediately and didn't bring it into the house for Sally to see. I left it just outside the front door,' says Stephen. 'I know it wasn't intentional, but the way Sally was feeling under the circumstances, it would have been too much for her to handle once the crowds went home.'

Sally remembers a call to another girlfriend.

'It was really awkward. We hadn't spoken in a few months and she immediately launched into telling me all about herself and her family. How was I going to interrupt her chit-chat to share my awful news? I eventually plucked up the courage, but she was so taken aback and upset by what she heard that I really wasn't sure how to react. My usual instinct would be to comfort her and tell her everything was going to be okay. But I couldn't do that now; nothing I said was going to make her feel any better and there were certainly no words she could offer up to soothe my pain.'

By the time Sally called her manager to let him know she wasn't going into work on the Monday, she could barely string a sentence together. 'The poor guy was left to interpret the news between my violent sobs.' She acknowledges how compassionate her workplace was to allow her almost six months of paid leave and great flexibility on her return.

During those first few days, after the initial news started to spread, the house was constantly filled with close friends who came over to show their support, bringing cakes, muffins and coffee with them, or simply leaving three-course meals on the doorstep.

'A lot of it ended up with our dog, Ollie, to be honest,' says Sally sheepishly. 'Neither Stephen nor I could manage to stomach much more than coffee at the time. I figured, why should I be enjoying food when my son would soon have even this basic pleasure taken away from him by this mystery disease?'

By Monday morning there were so many unknowns that Stephen oddly found himself thinking about cameras, video recorders and data storage. Normally he would have spent hours on the internet, researching models and obsessively hunting down the best deal, or negotiating just for fun; instead, he ordered online an IBM server with enormous storage capacity and automatic backups.

'I'd had a hard drive crash and lost a lot of photos a few weeks earlier; we weren't going to risk that ever happening again.'

Sally's brother showed up, carrying a new Sony HD video camera in his arms, soon after Stephen had returned from a trip to JB Hi-Fi, where he had just bought a top-of-the-range Canon HD video camera without even bothering to ask the price.

They both wanted to capture as many memories of Massimo as possible.

Chapter 4

ABOUT A BOY

Three state-of-the-art computer screens form a giant triptych on Stephen's antique desk. On the left screen, CNN runs silently in the background with breaking news alerts announcing hurricanes, missing planes and global market reports. In the centre, emails chime musically as they parachute into his crowded inbox every few minutes. On the right screen, real-time feeds update him on social media and business performance. At one end of his home office, standing 7 feet tall, is Gene – a faceless, inflatable astronaut, overseeing the constant comings and goings of the FedEx driver who visits the house on a daily basis.

Photos of Stephen's family line the walls, interspersed by framed Bachelor degrees in Planning and Design, Building, Computer Science and an MBA. One frame hangs empty, still awaiting the Master of Marketing Stephen had to cut short when Massimo became ill. To the left of a chesterfield sofa, a large mounted model of the XCOR Lynx spacecraft stands out among other planes and rockets. Ollie, the family's nine-year-old Rottweiler, pads in and out of the room, guarding his favourite spot under Stephen's desk.

'He was our first child,' says Stephen, giving him a pat on the head.

As soon as Massimo was born, he let out a hearty cry. It signalled to Sally and Stephen that they had a healthy baby and Stephen breathed a sigh of relief, only to be thrilled moments later when he heard the midwife saying, 'It's a boy!'

'I'd always wanted a son, so that brought a special smile to my face,' Stephen says. 'Within nanoseconds, life with our son flashed through my mind's eye. He'd be my assistant mechanic as we tinkered with cars on the weekend, and I would take each and every opportunity to teach him applied science from an early age. He would probably attend the same school as I did, only a few hundred metres walk from our home. And, of course, with a name like Massimo Damiani, he'd go on to be a Formula One World Champion for Ferrari,' he says jokingly.

'Stephen and I had already been married five years before we even started thinking about having a child,' says Sally.

It was Stephen who was getting clucky. Sally felt they should wait until the new business Eyre BioBotanics grew, wanting to be sure they would be financially secure, finish renovating their house, travel together a little more.

'I offered up a thousand reasons why it wasn't the right time to try for a baby,' she says.

But she succumbed to the idea, and a couple of months later, Sally was rushing up and down the aisles of Coles supermarket in Elsternwick on a Friday night, doing the shopping ahead of a weekend she planned to spend studying for an upcoming MBA exam.

'I threw a pregnancy test into the trolley, alongside some cotton tips, toothpaste and toilet paper – just in case.'

She woke early the next day and spent a peaceful hour in the kitchen, sipping coffee and reading the paper while Stephen slept in.

'I've always been a morning person. My parents were up at the crack of dawn when I was growing up – my father woke at 3 am most days to go and buy produce from the market. I have fond memories as a teenager of sharing an early morning coffee with him while we both watched the news on TV. To this day I love waking up before everyone else and enjoying the quiet as I prepare for the day ahead.'

When she finished her coffee, Sally grabbed the pregnancy test she'd bought the night before and made her way to the bathroom to have a shower. After she finished and brushed her hair, she casually glanced across at the white plastic stick. Two solid blue lines stared back at her. Could she be that lucky to have fallen pregnant after only two months of trying?

Sally raced out of the bathroom waving the pregnancy test above her head like a winning lottery ticket. She burst into the study to show Stephen, who was now up, coffee in hand, wading through a string of emails that had come in overnight.

'He was intensely focused on whatever was on his screen and barely noticed me, so I just put the test kit on the desk, right in front of him.'

Looking down to see the two blue lines, it took Stephen a few moments to realise what it was.

'You're pregnant?' Stephen was beaming from ear to ear.

Their life was about to change dramatically.

The house Dr Leah Kaminsky grew up in stands at the end of Stephen and Sally's street. She must have walked past what is now their home thousands of times through the years, heading either to or from the milk bar on the corner. The child of immigrant parents who had taken pride in bulldozing an old weatherboard to build their 1960s brick veneer three-bedroom dream home, she would feel sorry for the old ladies who lived alone in the rundown old cottages of the day. Stephen and Sally's home is one of those houses from the 1800s that were saved and have since been meticulously restored.

Dr Kaminsky's clinic is only a five-minute drive from the area. Even though Stephen and Sally had been patients there for a number of years, on the rare occasions they were sick they usually saw another doctor in the practice.

Now that Sally was pregnant she made an appointment for a routine antenatal visit. Her doctor happened to be on leave that day, so it was Leah who checked her blood pressure, weighed her, wrote out a form for blood screening and booked her in with an obstetrician. That was the first day Massimo came into Leah's world.

'Leah didn't waste time and booked me in for a foetal ultrasound the evening of my first appointment with her. The ultrasound confirmed that I was pregnant. As it was quite early in the pregnancy, all we saw was a little squiggly shape on the screen, earning Massimo his first nickname – Peanut. The radiologist estimated that Massimo would be due on 4 August 2008. Stephen joked that it would be great if the baby arrived late and was born on 08/08/08 – eight being a lucky number in Chinese culture, especially given the fact that the baby was conceived during a trip to Hong Kong a month earlier.'

Sally barely suffered from morning sickness. Her entire pregnancy went smoothly and she was at work all the way through, until a fortnight before her due date. Two days into her maternity leave, her waters broke in the middle of the night.

'Are you sure you haven't just wet the bed?' Stephen asked, because she was going to the bathroom several times a night.

'Don't be ridiculous!' She went searching for the number of the hospital.

The nurse on call insisted they come in, so Sally quickly packed a bag and jumped into the shower.

Stephen was on a strict diet and exercise program at the time, consisting of intensive interval and strength training coupled with five small protein-based meals a day. Each night before heading to bed, he prepared the ingredients for his morning omelette, chopping up bacon, onions, mushrooms, peppers, cheese and tomatoes. He always had everything ready in advance so that in the morning he could just throw the ingredients into a frying pan and cook it all up quickly. When Sally emerged from the shower at 2 am, the pungent smell of bacon and eggs greeted her as she opened the bathroom door. Stephen was standing at the kitchen bench munching on his omelette, a look of confusion and apprehension on his face.

'It was bizarre, but I didn't bother asking why he was eating an omelette at that hour. I think he was just confused. In his mind he thought we were going into hospital and would be back home later in the day.'

Several weeks earlier, Sally and Stephen had attended birthing classes. Each one ran for three hours, two evenings a week, and finding time in their schedules was a real challenge.

'The classes may as well have been called childbirth simulations, they dragged on for so long,' says Stephen. 'I must have been paying attention most of the time, though, because I seemed to know what was going on during the actual delivery. All of a sudden she started pushing and cursing at me – the midwife had already warned me about this transition phase. Not long after, in a tangle of hands, our newborn son came flying out, covered in slime.'

Their stay in hospital with Massimo was relatively uneventful. They cautiously bathed their little boy for the first time and Sally struggled with breast-feeding. A constant stream of guests filled the room with flowers and chocolates. But Stephen's mother, Hilda, who for years had longed for a grandchild, was quiet when Stephen brought her in to visit. She wasn't nearly as excited as they had expected her to be and repeatedly asked what the baby's name was. They would later discover she had Alzheimer's disease.

Four days later, Massimo was heading home to become the centre of this family's life. He was dressed in a designer outfit and strapped into his snazzy new Peg Perego convertible baby capsule, which Stephen had selected following one of his typically drawn-out research exercises.

'The drive home was terrifying,' says Sally. 'I couldn't come to terms with not having Massimo by my side, so I opted to sit in the back seat alongside him for the short ten-minute drive home from the hospital. When we pulled into our driveway on that chilly Saturday morning it was as though the enormity of bringing a new life into the world suddenly hit me all at once. It dawned on me that we were responsible for this little human being who was sleeping soundly in his capsule, breathing softly, oblivious to the panic that was unfolding around him. There was no nurse at the end of the call buzzer who could come and give me breast-feeding advice. Would my baby starve if I wasn't able to feed him properly? He was so tiny and delicate. I was bursting with love for this little person who we hardly knew, yet were so close to already, and this overwhelming feeling of adoration mixed with fear and anxiety culminated in my bursting into tears. When Stephen asked me what was wrong, all I could manage to say between sobs was, "I just love him so much, I don't want to break him." '

Sally and Stephen's dreams for Massimo were like those of most parents – they wanted to give their child the world, allow him to experience as much as possible, whether it was art, music, travel or sport. Stephen's mother was multi-lingual, so they planned for her to speak to Massimo in French; Stephen's father would sing to him in Italian. Sally's father would teach him Armenian, and of course their child would be a genius.

'We wanted Massimo to be able to choose his passion and not be forced to love something because of us,' says Sally.

Stephen agrees. 'I could never be a father who pushed my son down a preordained path. He would choose his own destiny and have my full support to realise his dreams.'

Stephen had grown up in a hard-working, post-war single-parent family. His mother had high ambitions for her son, hoping he would become a doctor.

'She wanted me to pursue the career she hadn't been able to and practised focused, incessant nagging,' which Stephen says backfired, pushing him away rather than inspiring him. As for his father: 'He lived for the day and was never around.'

Stephen is an affable guy, who speaks quickly and passionately, gesturing with his hands to emphasise important points he wants to get across. He stares at you through his red-framed glasses with a kind of half-smile, his eyebrows raised, as if to check whether or not you have really understood him.

Stephen's parents separated when he was still a baby.

'Dad was certainly not a good role model for family life,' he says, with more than a hint of disappointment in his voice. 'He moved on from us before my first birthday. Mum and I lived with my elderly grandmother, who died when I was twelve. My mother worked hard to send me to a good school and wanted me to have the opportunities she didn't have growing up in post-war Europe.

'I certainly wasn't an academic during my teens. There were too many distractions, and chalk and talk just wasn't the way I learned,' he says. 'I was always more of a hands-on techo kid. I loved pulling apart gadgets to find out how they worked. I learned more about DC current through diagnosing an electrical problem on a circuit board than by completing a series of text-book exercises. I grew up surrounded by computers, punch cards and floppy discs, which Mum would bring home from work when I was young.'

His parents' early separation meant Stephen grew up pretty much alone, with a sense of isolation always hovering in the background.

'I guess I learned at an early age to cope with solitude better than most. I didn't know any better.'

His father would make 'celebrity appearances' every few months to take them on a drive down the coast for the day. He came back into the picture a little more when he retired and his only son turned sixteen; together they would tinker on a classic car Stephen had bought with his own money to restore.

'I spent more time with him then than at any other time in my life. He wasn't one to throw his hands up in the air or give up on a tough practical task. He was methodical in diagnosing problems. If something blew up at home, he was never content to let someone else repair it until he had tried himself, even if it made the problem worse initially. He would always quote Thomas Edison – "Many of life's failures are people who did not realise how close they were to success when they gave up." I learned from him not to be afraid to fail. It's just a pity he wasn't around from an earlier age.'

Stephen had no intention of repeating his father's mistakes, instead seeing his roles as father to Massimo as those of counsellor, educator, facilitator and above all friend.

Once Massimo was born and the three of them began to settle into their new life, the anxiety of being new parents was slowly replaced by excitement for what the world had in store for their baby boy. Sally and Stephen were eager to get to know their son, anticipating the next cute thing he would do, whether it was the way he stretched out his arms and legs when they unswaddled him after a nap, or his habit of snuggling up to them after a feed, when he was drowsy. Despite sleepless nights, stinky nappies and even a bout of colic, the overwhelming feeling was that the world was right.

'We had become a family now that our baby was here.'

It was with great pride that they walked into Leah Kaminsky's office for Massimo's first check-up with a GP. It was particularly frantic at the clinic that day, however, so aside from offering perfunctory congratulations, Leah bypassed the chit-chat and went straight over to little Massimo.

'There is a fixed routine for examining a neonate head to toe,' she says. 'You need to completely undress the baby. First weigh them. Measure length and head circumference. Check the colour – pink is good, blue is definitely not. Palpate the fontanelles, look for symmetry of the face, insert a gloved finger into the mouth and use a torch to make sure there is no cleft palate, feel the tiny space between the skull bones, listen to the rapid lub-dub of the fledgling heart. Feel for clicks in the hips as you splay their legs out like a frog. The stepping reflex is always good for a laugh. I tell parents their baby is a genius who already knows how to walk. Leave the Moro reflex for last, because as you hold the baby's hands together and then let go, they will inevitably startle and let out a shriek. In essence, when you examine a baby, always look for something you don't want to find.'

Up until recently Leah had been in the habit of breathing a sigh of relief at the end of a normal examination and saying to the parents, 'Your child is perfect.' But lately she'd been thinking about this seemingly innocuous phrase and substituted it with the watered-down, 'Everything seems to be okay.'

She says, 'I remember as a young paediatric resident working at Prince of Wales Children's Hospital in Sydney, calling a senior consultant once when I had found some abnormality during an examination. He told me to check for two more imperfections – "Things come in threes with FLKs." In those days we used this coded term when the parents were present beside the crib, for a baby who in some way seemed unusual and warranted further investigation. FLK: Funny Looking Kid.'

Massimo had a 2 millimetre skin tag at the base of his spine. Leah remembered her professor's warning and so spent time scouring the baby's body for any other signs or anomalous structures. The rest of his examination was unremarkable, but to be on the safe side she referred them for an ultrasound, which revealed the unusual tethering at the base of his spinal cord, a malformation that would most likely need surgery further down the track. Stephen and Sally were devastated. Neither they nor Leah realised then that it was only the start of this little boy's journey into the world of the unknown.

One afternoon, among the chaos of friends making coffee in the kitchen and children playing in the lounge room, several days after Massimo's latest, fateful MRI scan and the series of agonising tests he had endured, Sally heard the home phone ring. Lifting Massimo up onto her hip, she answered it reluctantly, expecting to have to go through the whole terrible story again with yet another distraught friend.

'Hello. It's Rick Leventer here,' came the gentle voice at the other end of the line.

Sally handed Massimo over to one of her friends and raced into a quiet room, closing the door behind her.

'I have the first round of test results back,' the neurologist told her.

Sally was shocked. They hadn't been expecting any answers for a few weeks yet.

'All the investigations we did on Massimo have come back negative,' he told her.

Sally was stunned; bewildered by the news. This meant Massimo didn't actually have any of the nasty diseases they had been convinced were on the cards.

'How could that be?' she blurted out.

'Sally, this is a good thing,' Rick explained. 'All the conditions we've now ruled out have very bad outcomes.'

It took Sally a while to process this information. While she certainly didn't wish any of these illnesses on her son, she and Stephen had been certain that the MRI scan findings, together with Massimo's symptoms, pretty much sealed his fate. She had even begun to take some small comfort from the thought that at least knowing what disorder their child had would provide them with focus. It meant they could reach out to families they had already started reading about and start investigating the very early treatments being developed in clinical trials. The news that all of these nasty conditions had been ruled out came as a mixed blessing.

'With that phone call, all of those doors were slammed shut and we had once again fallen into the abyss of the unknown.'

Chapter 5

NEVER LET GO OF HOPE

Sally and Stephen went back to see Leah at the clinic on the Wednesday after Massimo's ominous MRI scan. Their world had been turned upside down.

'My receptionist, Annette, forewarned me this wasn't going to be a quick or easy visit. Stephen had called first thing that morning to tell her the news and book an appointment to see me. Annette was visibly shaken as she led the family into my room, not knowing what to say. Both Sally and Stephen looked pale and exhausted as they sat down in the upholstered chairs beside my desk. Sally was doing everything she could to hold it together. She is a quiet sort of person with a natural instinct to please others; always a smile on her face. That morning was no different; the smile was there, but her eyes betrayed any attempts to hide her pain. Stephen's hands were shaking as he spoke, debriefing me on the dramatic events of the previous few days.'

'"Massimo has a Leukodystrophy, but they don't know which type," he said. I stared at them blankly. Before I even had a chance to confess that I'd never heard of the term, Stephen was sharing mounds of information they had gleaned from the internet. I felt so awkward – here they were coming to me for professional advice, yet they already knew far more about the condition than I did. I figured it would just be a matter of a bit of reading on my behalf, catching up on the latest research on PubMed so I could guide them through the medical merry-go-round they found themselves on. Little did I know then that to this day Stephen and Sally would continue to be many steps ahead of me and many of my colleagues, despite their complete lack of any medical training.'

What was crystal clear from the outset was that neither Stephen nor Sally was ever going to accept there was simply no hope for their little boy. They hadn't gone to Leah for pity, sympathy or grief counselling; they were there to ask for help navigating the purgatory of their son's mystery illness. They weren't trying to become neurologists or geneticists, they just wanted to bring their knowledge up to a level where they could brainstorm options with the specialists and researchers who held the answers to their son's life in their hands.

'It was to be a journey that would turn my own

preconceived ideas of the doctor–patient power differential upside down,' Leah says. 'I spent most of that consultation trying to help Stephen and Sally prioritise what needed to be done first. They outlined three immediate objectives that day: diagnose Massimo; fix Massimo; give Massimo siblings.'

Christmas lunch was always a large affair for Sally's family, and was dominated by her mother's side of the family – her four older brothers and their nine children. On her father's side there were only two guests – his mother and brother. They were far more reserved. Anyone looking in through the dining-room window on Christmas Day 1993, at the giant Christmas tree, the dining-room table laden with fresh oysters, platters of meat and seafood, trays of fresh fruit and sweets, would have thought it was a happy, festive occasion. But things were different that Christmas. The families were sitting around speaking in hushed tones, rather than the usual heated shouting and full-bellied laughter.

'Instead of Mum firmly planted in the kitchen preparing all the salads, frying the prawns and marinating meat for the barbecue,' says Sally, 'she was sitting quietly among the guests.'

Her mother, who would have normally been dressed in a smart new pant suit purchased especially to mark the occasion, wore an ankle-length floral dressing gown that day. A shaved patch of scalp peeked out from between strands of her trademark thick, dark hair, which hung limply around her shoulders instead of being sculpted into its usual stylish bob.

Only two weeks earlier, Sally had taken a cup of coffee and the morning paper into her mother's room to begin their Sunday ritual of sharing a coffee and poring over the news and gossip together. Mrs Bakian mentioned that her right leg felt numb, but neither thought much of it.

'Then I remember her stumbling out of bed and falling to the floor. In her typical style, Mum brushed the event off and proceeded to get on with her day, even though she was dragging her leg a lot. She even went to work over the next couple of days, until she finally made an appointment to see our family GP on the Wednesday, who sent her straight to hospital.'

Sally still feels she doesn't know the full details of her mother's illness. Her family has always preferred to keep things private, or perhaps, more accurately, brushed under the carpet. At the time, her father, trying to protect Sally and her brother, told them that their mother was only out on special day leave for Christmas and would most likely need to stay in hospital for some time. Sally understood there was something wrong with her mother's brain and judging by the grave faces of all around, it was serious.

'It's funny, I thought I was really clever growing up. If you had seen my report cards at school you would have agreed, but it's only on reflection that I see how naive I was, accepting whatever I was told at face value, not questioning anything and not seeking more information.

I was more book smart than street smart. I simply didn't think to challenge and question. You didn't do that in my family.'

Sally drifted around the house, half-heartedly chatting to the guests while grabbing every opportunity to eavesdrop on any conversation concerning her mother.

'Could this be her last Christmas?' one aunt whispered.

'She'll never be able to walk again,' said an uncle.

Sally overheard her father discussing whether it would be more sensible to modify the house for a wheelchair, or sell the house and buy something more suitable for an invalid.

'I started to worry then. How was I going to be able to care for Mum, take on the work she did in the house and study for my senior year, all at the same time?'

A couple of weeks later her mother was discharged from hospital. She'd had a stroke and was told she would never be able to walk independently again. Sally spent the last few weeks of the summer holidays caring for her.

'One morning, Mum decided she wanted to try to walk without her walking frame. She got up from the couch and started taking tentative small steps. Once she'd reached the other side of the living room – about an eight-metre stretch in all – she announced that she would no longer be using any aids and there'd be no need for the wheelchair. From that moment on, she took control of her own destiny, dismissing the advice of the medical team. Not only did she start walking that day, she even returned to work after a few months.'

Twenty-one years later, Sally's mother runs around, with a minor limp – barely noticeable on a good day – the only hint that something was ever wrong.

'I didn't realise it at the time,' reflects Sally, 'but that experience taught me that you don't have to blindly accept an imposed fate. You need to challenge it until you are certain there are no other options and only then accept it and adapt. It showed me a person can do almost anything once they put their mind to it.'

'When we returned to the physiotherapist a week after Massimo's initial hospitalisation,' says Stephen, 'his motor skills had deteriorated so rapidly that she wheeled out something called a Jenx Giraffe chair.'

Stephen remembers feeling ill throughout the consultation. They were being shown equipment used for children who, in the main, had no hope of recovery from their illness.

'There was nothing rehabilitative about the Jenx chair. It was more a symbol to us that we needed to accept Massimo was going to deteriorate.'

The contraption had a wooden panel in the shape of a smiling giraffe glued to each side – the manufacturer's well-intentioned attempt to make it look child-friendly. It reminded Stephen of Darth Vader's suit.

'The click of the brace on Massimo's chair sounded like the helmet sealing around Anakin Skywalker's head just before you hear him take his first signature artificial breath as Darth Vader.'

And, sure enough, Massimo screamed in defiance as they strapped him in.

'It was as if he somehow knew he was being bolted into his fate – one he certainly didn't want to accept.'

In the weeks that followed, despite Massimo's deterioration, every test came back as normal. Sally and Stephen saw his neurologist, Rick Leventer, for a review in late August. He had already sent a copy of Massimo's MR imaging to his colleague Professor Marjo van der Knaap at VU University in the Netherlands, who is considered an expert in MRI pattern recognition for Leukodystrophies. He discussed all the results with Stephen and Sally and explained more about the various types of Leukodystrophy that had already been ruled out. This left them one step closer to flailing in the category of the 50 per cent of these disorders that remain genetically unclassified. In effect, undiagnosed.

'By this stage we were spending almost every minute of the day researching online and purchasing dozens of research papers. The possibility of not achieving a diagnosis, losing our son without knowing why and not being able to have other children was not acceptable,' says Stephen.

Stephen's disappointment that the results had not turned up a distinct diagnosis must have been outwardly obvious, as Rick reinforced to the couple that this was actually good news. Some of the conditions they had excluded were really nasty.

'It was then that I started throwing everything out on the table,' Stephen says. 'Stem cells, gene therapies, you name it – and the answers were always a hushed "no". Rick told us none of that would be possible without a diagnosis and he was absolutely correct.'

It was at this point that Stephen asked Rick, 'If it's genetic, don't you just get Massimo's genome – his complete DNA map – and line it up with our genomes and identify what is unique to him?'

'It's not as simple as that,' Rick replied.

If each letter of Massimo's sequenced genome was 1 centimetre by 1 centimetre, it would stretch to the moon and back 4.6 times. Human DNA – our genetic blueprint – comprises almost 30,000 genes and six billion letters of genetic coding. Stephen was suggesting they search for one or two of these letters.

Stephen looked at Rick's face and broke down. 'There's really no hope, is there?'

After several moments of silence, Rick turned to Stephen and said, 'Never let go of hope – there is always hope.'

Chapter 6

MISSION IMPOSSIBLE

Rick Leventer remembers the very first time he met the Damiani family, the day after Massimo's fateful MRI scan in Emergency.

'I wasn't on ward service that Friday but a colleague of mine needed the day off, so I agreed to cover him for the day.'

He was called down to the neurology ward on the sixth floor to help make sense of a child's MRI scan that was puzzling the staff.

'Massimo was in the first bed on the right, in a four-bed ward. His parents stood beside him looking devastated and shell-shocked. Their world was spinning out of control. I always try to give parents hope without being flippant about it. If I don't lose hope then neither should they, especially when it comes to an undiagnosed condition, because the prognosis may not always be as bad as they had initially thought. We just don't know.'

Rick would continue as Massimo's neurologist and become well acquainted with Stephen and Sally as time passed.

'I soon realised that the way Stephen gains control of a situation is via understanding the problem and its intricacies. He really challenged me initially, insisting that the "answer must be there". Even though back in those days he seemed off the wall, I had to admit that what he was saying about genetic technology made sense. In retrospect, we can all see he wasn't the slightest bit whacky; it was all coming. Stephen was pushing the envelope as a parent; he had reached the same level of understanding as most clinicians and geneticists. And that was what was truly unique – the knowledge he had and how he was prodding us all to do things we hadn't done before. He was just ahead of his time.'

The expression 'pushing the envelope' was coined in the 1950s, when early astronauts attempted to fly rocketplanes like the X-15 to the edge of space. The 'envelope' refers to the atmosphere surrounding Earth. To reach its edge was to reach space. Rick Leventer is no slouch himself when it comes to breaking through barriers. When he was at school he wanted to become a vet, but he missed out on a place at university by a few marks. He settled for medical school and took some time off to work on a kibbutz overseas after finishing his first year of studies. He planned to complete his medical degree and then go back and do veterinary training. He had it all mapped out – he would set himself up in two semi-detached houses and work as a vet on Mondays and Tuesdays, as a doctor on Thursdays and Fridays with Wednesdays off to play golf. Even up until five years ago he was still thinking of going back to apply for vet school.

His love for animals started when he was a kid, growing up in the Melbourne suburb of South Caulfield, not far from where Stephen Damiani spent his childhood years. Rick liked to play in the garden with insects, mice and lizards. He also built things, and was keen on taking apart mechanical objects to see how they worked. He got in trouble with his teachers for sometimes bringing his inventions or dismantled objects to school, including peeled golf balls, which would spontaneously disassemble on his desk as their rubber bands burst away. He spent a lot of time outside, and found it fascinating to try to figure out how things were made, pulling apart his toys and taking on projects with his dad to put them back together again. The two of them built a mouse cage and Rick continued to breed mice throughout his teenage years. He was given a set of golf clubs for a bar mitzvah present, but was far more interested in the long, thin box they came in, using it to house a family of local skinks he'd found.

Rick spent several years as a neurology research fellow in the United States, when he volunteered to be on the medical advisory board at the Lincoln Park Zoo in Chicago, observing annual check-ups for their gorillas and helping administer their tuberculosis tests.

How do you do a skin-prick test on an animal as large as a gorilla? 'With a lot of anaesthetic,' he says, laughing.

On his return to Melbourne, Rick was delighted that the Royal Children's Hospital had a long-term affiliation with Melbourne Zoo, located within walking distance from his clinic, across a leafy park. One evening Rick was called in there to give advice on a Sumatran tiger cub born with ataxia. It had poor muscle coordination, which gravely affected its ability to walk. The vets were perplexed and unable to come up with a diagnosis. Rick and his colleagues snuck their striped, furry patient into the hospital under cover, placing the little guy in an MRI scanner to see what was happening inside his brain. Unfortunately, they never found the diagnosis.

Rick always felt Stephen and Sally had faith in him. 'They knew I was on board, I just didn't have a mechanism at the time – neither funding nor manpower – for taking a genetic diagnosis any further. We all saw the promise of genomics, but had to temper Stephen's dreams with the reality of our limited resources.'

Looking back on it now that he is a father of two young children, Rick feels he has a deeper understanding of parents' anxieties. He is less dismissive of what he used to think of as small concerns, such as a child presenting with fever or lethargy. Through becoming a father, he feels he has learned more compassion for the parents of his young patients.

*

Once the initial salvo of tests came back negative, Rick suggested Massimo return to hospital for a couple of days in a further attempt to establish a diagnosis. This time Massimo was admitted to the neuroscience ward because 'things happen faster as an in-patient'. During this visit, the family were also introduced to a speech pathologist, occupational therapist and social worker who could offer support as his condition advanced.

'We were being educated on how to deal with the progressive loss of skills that was going to be the reality of our potentially short time with Massimo,' says Sally.

Aside from health professionals to assist with Massimo, the Damianis were also introduced to a local support group called Very Special Kids. They provide help to families caring for a child diagnosed with a life-threatening condition, offering both respite and end-of-life care.

'This was perhaps the most confronting thing of all,' says Stephen. 'In August, time had stopped. There were thousands of emails in my inbox and I hadn't bothered to read any that had to do with business for over two weeks. I remember sitting at my desk, unshaven and still in my pyjamas, the curtains drawn during business hours, as I looked up the Very Special Kids website. I had driven and walked past the Very Special Kids house thousands of times over the years without ever realising it was Melbourne's only hospice for children with life-threatening conditions. I had seen their huge pink piggy banks on trailers but only knew they were for some sort of fundraising. Now I was reading about the counselling, support and respite they provided to families who have a terminally ill child. I realised we had become one of those families.'

While Massimo lay in his hospital crib, a group of specialist metabolic physicians came to examine him top to toe, prodding his liver, feeling the size of his spleen, looking for unusual bone formation or strange facial features. Not an inch of the little guy was left unchecked.

'He was X-rayed, had ultrasounds, another horrific spinal tap and had more blood extracted from his tiny body than I thought would have been possible,' says Stephen. 'Nothing seemed to be straightforward or easy; even what should have been a simple blood test went horribly wrong. Massimo wailed uncontrollably, despite a topical anaesthetic being applied. The screaming was more out of pure fear than pain.'

Braced in Stephen's arms, Massimo endured three unsuccessful attempts to access a vein. Blood was spilling everywhere. Stephen fought hard to hold it together, sweating profusely and holding his breath. At times he closed his eyes to shut out the sight of Massimo writhing, tears streaming down his cheeks. Massimo screamed for ten minutes straight until his little voice was lost, reduced to a silent whimper. The moment enough blood had been collected Stephen jumped off the bed, pushing everyone aside as he passed Massimo to Sally. The child collapsed in her arms from exhaustion and Stephen raced out of the room into the corridor, visibly shaken and gasping for air. It took a few minutes to compose himself and he remembers everyone else leaving the room looking white from the experience. He didn't want his son to be tortured with tests in the little remaining time they had left together, but there was no choice if they were going to achieve a diagnosis.

This was just another step in their process of desensitisation, which had started earlier in the year and was about to be taken to the next level. Back in June 2009, during a routine ultrasound of Massimo's kidney, his ureter – the pipe connecting the kidney to the bladder – was seen to be dilated and open with fluid. This was a concerning finding, especially because Massimo only had one kidney, which raised questions about the stability of his bladder function. A urodynamic test was ordered, in which the bladder is filled with saline using a catheter and then filmed as it empties, checking for adequate function.

'It was an awful procedure which lasted thirty minutes, as the catheter insertion failed three times,' says Stephen. 'It felt like hours as we held Massimo down through his uncontrollable screams. It was horrible having to subject him to all this, but it seemed necessary for his long-term health. This was the first step in a long, drawn-out process, which would eventually go on to almost numb our sense of emotion. I don't think you ever fully recover from these experiences; you certainly never quite see the world in the same way again.'

The test showed that Massimo's bladder was working fine, but an additional renal scan was required to look at the blood supply, function and excretion of urine from his single kidney, as in his case an infection could prove life-threatening.

'Of course, Stephen being Stephen,' says Sally, 'he had already devised his own urodynamic test many months prior because of the single kidney. He calculated the volume of Massimo's bladder from an earlier ultrasound, which was approximately 22 millilitres, and reasoned that a wet nappy should weigh more in 22 gram multiples if his bladder was functioning correctly and completely emptying. He printed a spreadsheet and placed it next to the change table and bought a precision scale from eBay to weigh Massimo's nappies when they went on dry and when they were changed, giving us all detailed instructions. Sure enough, over the course of four weeks all of the full nappies were within a couple of grams of his model. He entered all the data onto his spreadsheet, worked out the supporting statistics and concluded there was no issue. I remember when he explained this to the first urologist we saw in the Spina Bifida Clinic and pulled out the spreadsheet and graphs, he nodded and said, "I have never seen this done before – very interesting." Like many clinicians and therapists who would go on to meet him over the years, he probably thought Stephen was a little over the top. Immersion is Stephen's way of taking control of problems at a practical level, to understand them thoroughly.'

Sadly, Massimo would soon have to endure far worse procedures.

*

'I held Massimo while he slept for two hours after that ordeal of the blood test, not wanting to put him down for fear of something else being done to him,' Sally says, her huge brown eyes welling up with tears. 'They always seemed to leave him alone when he was asleep. The following day, though, we went through the worst of it all – a skin biopsy.'

Sally assumed that Massimo would be anaesthetised or sedated beforehand, but instead only a topical numbing cream was applied. When they were led into a small examination room, she was asked to hold down Massimo's wrist and forearm, while a young doctor punctured his skin with an instrument that looked like an apple corer. He carved out a chunk of skin to be sent to the laboratory for analysis.

'I felt so conflicted,' says Sally. 'I knew Massimo needed to have these tests if we were ever going to diagnose him, but pinning him down while he screamed hysterically so the doctors and nurses could carry out their painful procedures made me feel like I was complicit in his suffering. As if it wasn't bad enough that I had made my son ill by passing on some hereditary illness, I was now torturing him in an attempt to find that defective gene.'

At a follow-up consultation with Rick they were told that neither the skin biopsy nor any of the other arduous tests had shed any more light on a diagnosis.

'One month had already passed since the master alarm sounded that night of his MRI scan,' says Stephen. Any further tests left that still might rule out various conditions and help narrow down the diagnosis were rapidly running out.

'Never in my life had I found myself in such a hopeless situation. I imagined this might be what it feels like to be on a plane about to crash. At some point your instincts accept the end is near. You can see the ground getting closer, the altimeter is spinning uncontrollably towards zero, but there is not enough time to pull up. You close your eyes and it's all over in a flash. In our case, though, we couldn't see the end clearly – was it weeks, months, years or decades away?

'We started planning for every possible future outcome, but could really only live for the day. It was tough, very tough; I felt like I was going crazy. I am a planner and don't cope well with uncertainty. The only way I could manage was to throw everything behind a diagnosis, and despite knowing this was a giant gamble, I had to take a leap of faith. I needed to understand why this was happening. If we were ever going to develop a treatment one day, we needed a diagnosis. In theory, it was possible and I simply wasn't going to give up until I had one. That was a commitment I made to my son.'

From around mid-August, after the initial three weeks of crisis, Stephen's mind went back to that 'Cracking the Code' edition of *Time* magazine he had read years before while grounded on that plane at Charles de Gaulle Airport. He remembered how captivated he had been with the Collins and Venter promise of a paradigm shift in medicine through the successful mapping of the human genome, deciphering the very basic code of life.

Stephen learned that the units that make up DNA are called nucleotides, and four of them – adenine, thymine, cytosine and guanine – are arranged together in strings. Three billion pairs of these strings make up our DNA blueprint called a genome. As he recalled the old article, Stephen assumed this historic feat that would change medicine forever had surely become a mainstream clinical reality by now.

Stephen says he always felt that identifying Massimo's broken gene, in theory at least, wasn't as complicated as many people thought, but now admits he was somewhat optimistic and naive.

'Don't you just align Massimo's genome with mine and Sally's, and run it through a set of complex differential algorithms on an IBM Watson super computer to find a variation unique in him? It's just lots of data, statistical analysis and brute force computing power. We have peta-flops of computing power these days. How hard can it be?'

Diagnose Massimo. Give Massimo siblings. These were priorities for Sally and Stephen. Leah managed to get them an appointment to see a clinical geneticist within weeks instead of months to discuss the options for testing and screening for a future pregnancy. A couple of hours after the review meeting with Rick, Stephen and Sally sat in the overflowing public obstetrics and genetics clinic at the Royal Women's Hospital. Eventually, they were called into a tiny consultation room, where a clinical genetics fellow asked them a series of questions about their ethnicities and any family history of illness. She sketched out a family tree, using circles to represent females and squares for males. Eventually her supervisor, an associate professor of genetics, came in and sat down. He skimmed Massimo's medical record and directed some teaching comments at the clinical genetics fellow, then scribbled a few notes into the file.

'Yes, you probably have a one in four chance of this happening again. That is, if the condition is recessive. We just don't know.' The professor sat in his chair, hands firmly planted in his pockets.

Stephen and Sally already knew a recessive condition generally does not have any effect unless the child inherits a faulty gene from each parent. They had been researching relentlessly many aspects of genetics, wanting to come prepared for the meeting.

They were working to a crisis timeframe and asked about every possible testing and screening scenario they could think of to expedite the process, based on their rudimentary knowledge of genetics at the time.

'The clinical geneticist told us we first needed to better understand what was wrong with Massimo, and only then could they proceed with testing specific genes. We felt as though the process couldn't keep up with Massimo's needs,' says Stephen. 'We needed to be able to test everything simultaneously, to get an answer as quickly as possible. I didn't feel as though we were going to be able to do that, testing one or only a few genes at a time. If we followed the status quo, it could take a decade to achieve a diagnosis, and Massimo didn't have that sort of time. What we needed was a shotgun approach, testing all 30,000 genes at once. Free from all financial limitations, we needed to be committed to doing whatever was necessary – right here and now – to figure out the cause of our son's condition.'

The associate professor shrugged his shoulders. 'Unfortunately, you may never find the gene causing the disease because almost half of these conditions remain undiagnosed.'

He asked if they had more questions, then stood up to signal the consultation had come to an end.

Stephen left the room questioning the approach and feeling despondent. There seemed to be a general acceptance there was a high likelihood Stephen and Sally may never get a diagnosis.

'There was no decision tree or "big animal chart" of "we are here and these are all of the possible steps we are going to go through to identify the cause of this condition right through to a diagnosis,"' Stephen says. 'We had already done so much research prior to the meeting and went in hoping there was something we might have overlooked and that more could be done. Unfortunately, we hadn't missed anything. Was there really nothing else out there?'

The clock for Massimo was ticking. With no clear roadmap or timeframe for the steps they might take to reach a diagnosis, Stephen and Sally left the clinic with an ever-diminishing sense of hope.

*

Massimo's condition continued to deteriorate rapidly. He began choking on both food and water, lost all of his vocabulary, and was no longer able to crawl or sit.

'He looked sick and weak, but worst of all he seemed frightened,' says Stephen. 'And although no one ever said so, I don't think any of us really expected him to see much of 2010.'

He was being managed by a large team of clinicians, each one attending to a different aspect of his illness. Few of the medical professionals and internet support groups were all that encouraging, and with fair reason. The prognosis for infant-onset Leukodystrophies is grim: in the order of months to several years at best. The consensus continued to be: 'Take your son home and enjoy whatever little time you have left with him.'

But they didn't know what a stubborn guy Stephen can be. Perhaps it runs in his genes, as his father comes from the Abruzzo in Italy. The Abruzzese have a reputation for being hard-headed, or *testa dura*. Rocky Marciano, the only World Heavyweight Champion to go undefeated throughout his career, was of Abruzzese heritage.

'If we had accepted all the advice and opinions we were given from around the world, we wouldn't be where we are today,' Stephen says. 'I fully appreciated that the chances of achieving a diagnosis with only one affected child were slim at best. However, I couldn't look in the mirror and tell myself we had done anything and everything possible to diagnose and maybe save our little boy. I just wasn't ready to accept this fate without testing the theory of cracking the code using our genomes. I had to exhaust this option before I could have a clear conscience. Even if the chances were one in six billion, it was better than none in six billion.'

They went back to see Leah at the clinic. She suggested they get in touch with a counsellor, to help support them through their sudden plummet into the daunting maze of the medical world. For the first few weeks Sally seemed to be keeping it together emotionally; far more than Stephen. Perhaps because he was the one who tended to speak up during consultations, he was also the one tearing up and breaking down. Or maybe it was because he grasped the technology, and understood the monumental scale of the challenge to diagnose Massimo before most. Stephen never thought achieving the diagnosis was going to be impossible. In fact, he was convinced the technologies to sequence, analyse and identify a single genetic variation all existed and were ready to be put to the test. The challenge was going to be bringing together the funding and people to make it happen for his son.

Stephen cast his mind back to the start of perhaps one of the most extraordinary periods of advancement in science, technology and engineering: the 1960s space race, President Kennedy's promise to the American people to land a man on the moon and return him safely to Earth before the end of the decade.

'Like any small boy, I was always fascinated with aviation, aerospace and all things pointy and fast,' says Stephen. 'I remember staying up late to watch the first space shuttle launch when I was in Year 3, and I was in awe from that point. The space program always seemed to be at the cutting edge – going further, faster, higher and into new frontiers with every step. It was an era when science was driven by imagination, and anything was possible. If we were to achieve a diagnosis we needed to free the science. Rather than be hindered by the ivory-tower ethics of secondary findings, bureaucracy and budgets, researchers needed to be inspired by imagination without constraint.'

Stephen says, 'The Apollo program may have been politically motivated, to some degree, but it united a nation to achieve a common goal and the results were nothing short of spectacular. Massimo needed his own Apollo program.'

They called it Mission Massimo, and failure was not an option.

When Jerry Bostick, Flight Dynamics Officer on the Apollo 13 mission, was asked if people at Mission Control were frantic with fear when the astronauts' lives were in danger, he answered, 'No. When bad things happened, we just calmly laid out all the options, and failure was not one of them. We never panicked, and we never gave up on finding a solution.'

Realising the enormity of their challenge, Stephen sketched out what was to form the basis of Mission Massimo, an audacious plan to diagnose and eventually develop a treatment for his son. It was a Venn diagram that essentially mapped out the strategic division of labour between him and Sally: Diagnose / Treat / Manage.

This approach allowed Stephen to focus his efforts on achieving a diagnosis and eventually the development of a therapy. It gave Sally room to concentrate on affording Massimo the best quality of life. While each of them threw themselves into the task at hand, they dealt with the situation in their own unique way.

Sally put all her energy into finding the right team of therapists to help care for Massimo. She spent countless hours ringing myriad speech therapists, occupational therapists and physiotherapists.

'Leukodystrophy is so rare that finding people who knew what it was and understood Massimo's specific needs was almost impossible,' she says. 'It was essentially a process of trial and error, calling or visiting therapist after therapist in between all our other appointments.'

Overwhelmed by the real possibility she would soon lose her son, Sally internalised her pain, maintaining a focus on Massimo to distract herself during the day. The nights were different though. 'Each night, as I put Massimo to bed, I wondered how many more opportunities I would have to do this. What would the last time be like?'

After half-heartedly slapping dinner together, Sally would assume her position on the opposite end of the couch to Stephen, each of them searching the internet for more information.

'While Stephen was devouring the scientific papers, I would obsessively look for anything about other families with a child with Leukodystrophy. How did they care for their kids? What medications did they use to manage symptoms? What kind of therapy helped them?'

Stephen, wired on dozens of coffees during those few

weeks as he researched diagnostic and treatment options, as well as planning modifications to their house to make Massimo more comfortable, would end up drinking himself to sleep most evenings.

'The moment Massimo went to bed, the red wine came out and I was knocking back one or two bottles every night. The comedy *30 Rock* would be on in the background to distract me from the situation, but I always had two laptops running simultaneously. I hardly slept, but when I did I had a recurring nightmare. I was reading a eulogy at Massimo's funeral, in a room packed with people, and the music playing was a baby song we always sang to him:

'Head, shoulders, knees and toes, knees and toes
Head, shoulders, knees and toes, knees and toes
and eyes and ears and mouth and nose,
Head, shoulders, knees and toes, knees and toes.'

Chapter 7

THE SECRET MISSION

Stephen and Sally follow in the footsteps of extraordinary parents such as Augusto and Michaela Odone, whose story inspired the 1992 film *Lorenzo's Oil*, starring Nick Nolte and Susan Sarandon. In 1984, Augusto, an economist for the World Bank, was told the news that his son, Lorenzo, six years old at the time, suffered from a rare, crippling type of Leukodystrophy called Adrenoleukodystrophy. Like the Damiani family, they were given little hope for their boy, who would gradually become blind, mute and deaf, as well as paralysed.

In those days, most children with Adrenoleukodystrophy died within two years of the onset of symptoms. The Odones refused to accept this dire prognosis, and fought to find a treatment for Lorenzo. With no medical background, and well before the age of the internet, they spent endless hours in the National Institutes of Health library, exhaustively trawling through research papers. They often clashed with the medical profession, as well as parents of children with similar conditions, who warned them that with no formal training it would be impossible for them to find a cure. Doctors believed that laypeople like the Odones had no way of understanding the specialised medical literature necessary to come up with an effective treatment.

Despite the scepticism, Augusto and Michaela developed a derivative of olive and rapeseed oil, reducing levels of specific fatty acids that build up in children with Adrenoleukodystrophy, who are unable to process them naturally. The formula was made by a retired scientist at Croda in the United Kingdom, who mixed oleic and erucic acids together. It became known as 'Lorenzo's Oil'. Although subsequently shown to work best only during the early stages of the disease, this mixture helped to prolong Lorenzo's life. He died in 2008, at the age of thirty. The Odones also established an organisation, the Myelin Project, to help promote research on Adrenoleukodystrophy and other similar myelin disorders.

Just like Sally, Michaela Odone was determined not to give up on her gravely ill son. Both mothers preserved their son's dignity by devising individualised means of communication – the blinking of eyelids to indicate yes and no by Lorenzo, and pointing to pictures on an iPad for Massimo.

Showing the same determination as Augusto Odone, Stephen was committed to finding a diagnosis for his son.

In early September 2009 he contacted a company on the East Coast of the United States that offered whole exome and genome sequencing. The human genome consists of three billion base pairs of nucleotides. But only a small percentage of those letters are actually translated into proteins. The exome consists of all the exons, which are the coding portions of genes. The term is derived from "EXpressed regiON", since these are the regions that get translated, or expressed as proteins. The exome forms only 1 per cent of the genome, but is thought to harbour around 85 per cent of all mutations which have a huge impact on disease. Although it seemed they might be able to perform this exercise, the cost in late 2009 to have a single exome sequenced was around US$15,000, and a whole genome was closer to US$100,000 plus analysis fees. They needed to sequence three and analyse them simultaneously, which was not an available commercial service being offered at the time.

Sally and Stephen returned to the Royal Women's Hospital to proceed with genetic testing for two conditions that had been raised as possibilities by Professor Marjo van der Knaap. Dr George McGillivray, a clinical geneticist, who had a special interest in neurological conditions, was to order tests for two types of Leukodystrophy that could only be performed overseas. The first was a condition known as Pelizaeus Merzbacher Disease, caused by mutations in the PLP1 or GJC2 genes, being tested at Nemours Alfred I. duPont Hospital for Children in Wilmington, Delaware, in the United States. The second newly described condition, known as Hypomyelination and Congenital Cataract, caused by mutations in the FAM126A gene, was only being tested in a research environment at the Giannina Gaslini Institute, in Genova, Italy.

Sally and Stephen had taken Massimo along with them and he slept contentedly in his stroller as they sat in the waiting room. Surrounded by pregnant women and their partners, by chance Sally bumped into an old friend, who excitedly told her she was expecting twins.

'Then she asked why we were at the hospital. I just couldn't answer. I started shaking on the spot, tears streaming down my face. Thankfully, Stephen jumped in and explained our situation.'

When they were called in, Dr McGillivray and his colleague Kate Pope, a genetic counsellor, introduced themselves and went through the same initial history-taking as the previous geneticist they had seen – a brief overview of inheritance patterns, the usual queries about family, drawing the circles and boxes that denote a family tree.

'We listened and waited patiently,' says Stephen, 'but as soon as we were given the opportunity to speak, a lot of questions came flooding out.'

Stephen put the idea of whole-genome sequencing on the table at this consultation. However, it was still considered to yield too much data to be meaningful, which also meant it would be extremely difficult to analyse and interpret, especially for only a single affected patient.

'I sensed Stephen's frustration that the human genome was not yet a clinical reality, but he didn't push the subject further,' says Sally. 'We were told that we were miles ahead of where most people would be in the same situation; that in a short six weeks we had covered ground that would normally have taken twelve to eighteen months.'

It should have been a comforting piece of information; instead, the Damianis were dismayed that there were people out there enduring this diagnostic odyssey and going through it all for so much longer.

'We discussed the case of a patient who had recently been diagnosed with a rare genetic condition at the age of thirteen,' says Stephen. 'Our hearts sank right there in the consulting room. Massimo didn't have thirteen years – at this stage he was going to be lucky to have thirteen months.'

After all their struggles to find a diagnosis for Massimo – endless hours over the previous month spent in hospital wards, clinics, doctors' offices, physiotherapists; the days and nights at home trawling the internet for possible clues to a diagnosis – Sally and Stephen decided they needed to restore a little normality in their lives. It was time to think about extending their small family. Moreover, they wanted Massimo to have siblings to love him, and for them to have the chance to meet each other before the inevitable happened. It was a glimmer of hope.

Through Sally and Stephen's experiences with genetic counselling, they understood they had no way of knowing if their next child would be born with exactly the same genetic illness as Massimo.

'We weren't prepared to risk having another child without a confirmed diagnosis,' says Stephen. 'The options available to grow our family safely were pretty limited. We could hold off and see if we got a diagnosis in Massimo, but with each salvo of tests coming back negative the chances of this weren't looking good in the near term. Waiting just wasn't an option either. Watching the dramatic rate at which Massimo was losing skills and becoming weaker meant his condition was following the tragic path of an infant-onset Leukodystrophy, where life expectancy is typically under five years. We were determined that any future siblings were going to be born within his lifetime. We wanted his future siblings to know Massimo as more than a framed picture on the wall.'

Massimo's devastating condition was something they were not willing to risk replicating if they were to have more children. An option available to them was to use an egg or sperm donor. At the time, the consensus was that they were quite possibly dealing with a disease caused by mutations in mitochondrial genes – a defect in the minuscule energy-producing machinery within each cell. Some of the estimated 30,000 genes in the human genome are located in the mitochondria, rather than on chromosomes within the cell's nucleus.

The genes found within the mitochondria contain the DNA that codes for the production of many of the important enzymes that drive the biochemical reactions to produce the body's source of energy: a chemical called ATP (adenosine triphosphate). The cells in the body, especially in organs such as the brain, cannot function normally unless they are receiving a constant supply of energy. In humans, mitochondrial DNA is inherited almost exclusively from the maternal side, so the greatest risk-reducing option would be to seek an egg donor.

They considered asking friends, but in their home state of Victoria it is recommended that any woman who acts as a donor needs to have finished having her family and preferably be over thirty-five years of age.

'This pretty much ruled out all of our friends, who were in the process of building their families,' says Sally. 'Besides, when we discussed egg donation in a general sense, it seemed to make everyone pretty uncomfortable. We did consider adoption, but a quick bit of research revealed the lengthy waiting periods involved, so we ruled it out early on. It was through this process of deduction that we arrived at needing an egg donor to assist us in growing our family and making sure Massimo would have siblings.'

Sally and Stephen didn't want to waste any time, so they decided to proceed immediately with donor IVF, in parallel to pursuing further serious research into genome sequencing to help diagnose Massimo. In early September 2009 they returned to see Leah, requesting a referral to see a top fertility specialist at Melbourne IVF. Leah picked up the phone immediately to arrange an appointment, but was told there was a six-month waiting list. Undaunted, she convinced the receptionist to squeeze Sally and Stephen in the following morning. Leah only found out much later that Stephen and Sally had nicknamed her Jack Bauer, the star of the TV series *24*, because of her chutzpah and ability to bulldoze her way past anyone in order to get the Damianis the urgent appointments they needed within twenty-four hours.

'I'm sure to this day,' says Leah, laughing, 'that some medical receptionists still tremble when they hear my voice on the other end of the phone, knowing I will torture them with endless hassling until they succumb and cough up a time slot for Stephen and Sally's family.'

Infertility was not something the couple had given much thought to prior to Massimo being diagnosed with Leukodystrophy. They had several friends who had undergone IVF and through Sally's mothers' group she met several more women who underwent IVF to conceive their children. 'Seeing all of this around me,' Sally says, 'made me grateful that Stephen and I conceived Massimo with relative ease, and that I was able to carry him to term without any complications.'

Nor had she ever really thought much about how many children she wanted. 'Stephen was an only child and I was one of two; neither of us being from huge families, a large family was never in sight. I enjoyed the companionship of my brother growing up and I always felt as though Stephen seemed a bit lonely being an only child, so I guess I assumed that we would have at least two children.'

Eventually, after all their deliberations, they decided a paid egg donor would be the fastest option, and would mean not having to worry about having any awkwardness afterwards with someone close. The irony was, however, that in Sally and Stephen's home state of Victoria paying for an egg donor is unlawful; you need to advertise and hope some altruistic woman will read your call for help. Stephen flicked through the pages of a local parents' magazine called *Melbourne's Child*. To his dismay, an entire page was filled with classified ads along the lines of 'Egg Donor Angel Needed to Start a Loving Family', or the heart-wrenching 'We are looking for a kind-hearted, generous Angel to donate her eggs. After three miscarriages we are begging you to help us with the greatest gift of life. All travel and medical expenses will be reimbursed.' Each ad, pleading for a woman to donate an egg, was summarily followed by the official government blurb that it is compulsory to include: 'This advertisement has been approved by the Victorian Minister for Health, as required by s.40 of the Human Tissue Act 1982 (Vic).'

By mid-September, Stephen sat at his desk feeling completely exhausted. 'Trying to organise IVF during that same period was honestly as big a feat to me as searching for a diagnosis for Massimo – where on earth to go, how to make it happen before we lost him? Waiting for someone to donate out of the goodness of their heart was going to take too long; Massimo simply didn't have that sort of time.'

'The lack of a diagnosis,' says Sally, 'constantly meant we had to jump extra hurdles, even when it came to something as natural as wanting to give Massimo a brother or sister.'

It soon became obvious that Stephen and Sally would have to search for a paid egg donor from overseas. Their options were to look to Greece, South Africa or the United States. The first two countries only allowed anonymous donors to participate in their programs, so Sally and Stephen opted for an American company. It was vital to them to have the option to be able to keep in contact with the egg donor and introduce her to their child at some point down the track, as she would always form part of their biological heritage.

As many as 60,000 children conceived through sperm donation have grown up in Australia with no idea of their paternal biological heritage and little hope of finding out. During the 1980s donors were recruited with the promise their identity and medical history would remain anonymous. Donor conception was an emerging area of medicine, at the cross-roads of ethics and science, which lay outside the law. Protecting the anonymity of donors overshadowed the rights of the conceived children.

In May 2011, Narelle Grech, a social worker from Melbourne, was diagnosed with advanced stage-four bowel cancer. The doctors immediately asked if there was a history of the disease in her family. She had been conceived through donation at the now defunct Prince Henry's Hospital and spent half her life searching in vain for the man known only by his donor code – T5. If she had known there was a potential risk of bowel cancer she could have taken a simple genetic screening test and caught it early. In February 2013, she finally met the sperm donor and discovered she also had eight half-siblings from the same donor. Narelle Grech passed away on 26 March 2013 at the age of thirty.

'I searched the internet and finally connected with a company called Donor SOURCE in the US,' says Stephen. 'It was daunting being able to scroll through criteria such as preferences for eye and hair colour, height, blood type, race, ethnicity and level of education, but it was an incredible relief just to be able to get on with it and not be concerned about other people's opinions. We already had so much else to worry about.'

Donor SOURCE's website advises potential parents that 'selecting an egg is one of the hardest decisions you'll ever face. It is important to think about what qualities mean the most to you and your partner.' Stephen and Sally sifted through a catalogue of donors designated by numbers rather than names, as if they were screening applicants for some key corporate executive position with only anonymous CVs at hand.

'It felt cold and clinical,' he says. 'From the start we had to make all sorts of choices that would potentially have enormous impact down the track – such as, should we choose a donor with the same blood type as Sally? At the time, we didn't want our next child to suddenly discover that their blood type wasn't compatible with ours and figure out that they weren't 100 per cent biologically related to their parents. We always wanted the child to know about their biological heritage and meet the donor but we also needed to be sure "the time to tell" was right for the child and it would come from us.'

'Many nights were spent discussing the pros and cons of our decision,' says Sally. 'What could potentially go wrong during the process? And would the whole thing be a secret? If not, then when would we tell our child the truth? What would we say to our friends and family? If we told everyone from the outset, what would happen if our child overheard others talking about him or her? How would they feel? Would they be picked on at school? Fast forward fifteen years, and a surly teenager lashes out in the heat of an argument and tells me I am not his/her real mother anyway. Would I be able to cope with that?'

They decided early on that shrouding things in secrecy would not only be futile, but counter-productive. They wanted their child to know that they had used an egg donor as soon as they were old enough to understand. Besides, they were beginning to learn the hard way, with several of their own family members not even acknowledging Massimo's illness, that genes alone don't make a family.

'When trying to narrow down what specific qualities we were looking for in a donor,' says Stephen, 'we initially preferred to find someone whose physical characteristics matched our own, preferably with a European genetic heritage, because we wanted to be able to tell our child about the donor in our own time, when he or she was ready. We didn't want them to find out accidentally, through a third party who questioned how two parents with olive complexions, brown eyes and dark hair could have a blue-eyed, blond-haired baby.'

As Sally's days were spent attending to Massimo's care needs, Stephen was the main driver of the process, trawling through the database of potential donors, narrowing the list down to a more manageable number that Sally could peruse when Massimo was sleeping.

'It took me a few days to come to terms with the process,' he says. 'Browsing through sheet after sheet of young women, one of whom was our potential donor, felt so impersonal. We were basically making one of the most important decisions of our lives via an online catalogue.'

They selected a potential donor based in Seattle, who had never had children or been an egg donor before. This was an advantage in Stephen's and Sally's minds, because they wanted, if possible, to avoid their next child having to deal with the emotional challenge of not only losing their brother at a young age, but of having multiple genetic half-siblings.

They contacted Donor SOURCE to ask for more information on the donor, and an initial teleconference call was set up within two weeks. The donor, a twenty-nine-year-old woman called Melinda, interviewed Stephen first in order to feel comfortable knowing who the biological father would be. She was accompanied by a case manager and asked some general questions, such as what they enjoyed doing as a family, how they celebrated Christmas and how much time they tended to spend together. Family was very important to her and that was a big plus for Stephen and Sally.

'I told her our situation, explaining that our son had a rare undiagnosed form of Leukodystrophy that meant it was highly likely he was going to die within the next twelve months. If we were to have any more children naturally it would mean a one in four chance of them inheriting the same fatal genetic disease as Massimo. The call lasted ten minutes and it felt like a legal settlement meeting, with the case manager coordinating it as a Q and A rather than a three-way conversation. I certainly wasn't the one in the power seat; it was Melinda interviewing me.'

Stephen came off the call certain he'd screwed up. It had been an intense two months since Massimo's fateful MRI scan result. He was so anxious and fatigued that he wasn't sure if what he'd been saying might have sounded like complete nonsense. To his delight they heard back from Donor SOURCE within twenty-four hours that Melinda was willing to be their egg donor. The reason she had signed up to be a donor in the first place was because she wanted to help people in some meaningful way. She had not had any children as yet, nor had she donated to any other families; in fact, she had been on the verge of removing herself from the register when she heard Massimo's story. She was so deeply moved that she had chosen to help Stephen and Sally have another child.

Stephen and Sally were then contacted by Seattle Reproductive Medicine, located in Melinda's home town. They were advised that all parties would have to undergo strict protocols, including drug screening, broad genetic testing and psychological counselling. From there, both women were started on separate medical protocols to synchronise their cycles for a successful egg transfer: Melinda was given hormones to produce an excess of eggs and Sally injections into her belly to prepare her womb for the implantation of an embryo. They set a date for the egg retrieval, hoping to maximise their chances of success by undergoing what was referred to as a fresh transfer – an embryo transferred before it is frozen.

By the second week of December, they were booked to leave for the United States. Stephen was scheduled to fly out three days earlier than Sally to start the IVF process, but also because he wanted to ensure they were on separate flights.

'If the plane went down with both of us on-board, what was going to happen to Massimo? Before we left, we drew up all our wills and cascading powers of attorney. We both flew on the Qantas Nancy Bird Walton from Melbourne to Los Angeles. I was excited to be flying on the A380 Airbus for the first time, although the check-in staff made me feel a little apprehensive when they jokingly referred to the aircraft as the "Scarebus". I was fortunate enough to fly on the upper deck, overlooking the port wing and its giant Rolls-Royce Trent 900 engines. Eleven months later, the Nancy Bird Walton's inboard port engine, which I had been sitting 10 metres away from, exploded shortly after take-off from Singapore.'

Despite being with 500 other passengers on the world's

largest commercial aircraft, it was the first time in five months Stephen felt as if he had some privacy.

'This should have been a flight where I enjoyed a few drinks and snuck in some uninterrupted sleep. However, it was the most apprehensive I have ever been on a flight, given the circumstances. I had stopped drinking over the preceding two weeks; was having daily saunas; drinking plenty of water and forcing myself to go to the gym and run regularly. As a consequence of this detox I couldn't enjoy a glass of wine, or take anything to help me sleep. I wanted to make sure my "chaps" were fighting fit and ready for their mission in Seattle.'

Stephen arrived in the United States just a couple of weeks before Christmas.

'Entering LAX arrivals hall, after a long-haul flight across the Pacific, is always a fun experience. The place was heaving with people. I must have looked like death going through Customs, and was dreading the inevitable questions at passport control – "What's your business in the United States?" What was I going to say? In the end, I just blurted out the truth: "I'm here for IVF because my son in Australia is dying and I don't know why." I am not sure what the Customs officer thought, but there was no second question. He just handed me back my passport and let me go straight through, calling out "Next".'

Unfortunately, Stephen's bag didn't arrive with him. He was told it was still in Melbourne, but would be 'expedited' to Seattle the following day. 'It was the peak of summer back home and all I had to wear was a paper-thin shirt and cabin suit from the plane. I arrived at the hotel and freshened up after twenty-four hours of travelling, and then headed downstairs. I ended up walking briskly down Eighth Avenue, shivering from the cold, and to top it off dropped my iPhone and smashed the screen. What more could go wrong? Was it an omen? I went straight into Nordstrom, the first store I could find, and bought a warm jacket.'

Three days later, on a frosty Sunday morning, he caught a cab from his hotel to Seattle Reproductive Medicine, on the shores of Lake Union.

'It was a yellow Ford Crown Victoria. The upholstery was filthy and the driver, who reeked of smoke, was talking on his phone the entire way. I felt nervous thinking I'd come this far and might not make it the final mile in one piece. He eventually dropped me in front of a concrete office block, in what felt like the middle of a ghost town. It was 8 am and there wasn't a soul in sight.'

Stephen pressed the buzzer at the front doors. A tinny voice came over the intercom, telling him to enter and take the glass elevator up to the third floor. A man in blue scrubs met him in the lift foyer and gestured for him to follow. Stephen was led to a small room in which there was a brown leather couch, TV with remote control and a few well-used magazines. He was handed a specimen bag and jar.

'When you finish, put it here.' The assistant pointed to a 20 by 20 centimetre stainless steel door in the wall. He told him to press a buzzer, and the bag and jar would be taken.

'I turned on the TV and sat on the couch for a moment wishing I had a glass of red to romance myself. It was all so impersonal, but for the first time in five months, I felt a sense of relief that we had made it all happen.'

When he had finished, he walked out into an empty corridor and took the lift downstairs again. By 8.45 am he was back outside on Galer Street. He sighed, relieved he'd completed his part of the mission. It was so cold he could see his breath. He walked across Westlake Avenue into an inviting warm Starbucks to escape the cold.

'Seattle is the home of Starbucks. I asked for a Tall Caramel Macchiato. I figured "when in Rome".'

Strolling along Westlake Avenue, warming his hands on the cup, he looked up and saw the Space Needle, the lofty landmark of Seattle, on his right, Lake Union to his left. He passed a sign for Kenmore Air, a sea-plane charter company, and stopped to take a photo. Then he hailed another yellow cab – this time a clean Toyota Prius – back to the hotel.

The following day, Stephen flew out to San Francisco for a pre-arranged meeting at the airport café with the founder of a genetic testing start-up company. In the course of their IVF cycle, Stephen and Sally had been offered a new pre-conception genetic test in the United States that screened for over a hundred devastating genetic diseases through a simple saliva sample, and it only cost a few hundred dollars. Results could be delivered within two weeks. Up until then there hadn't been anything available at a reasonable price with such a quick turnaround in Australia. The meeting lasted half an hour and ended with Stephen proposing to launch the test back home, in order to help prevent these terrible conditions from occurring. They parted with a handshake agreement for Stephen to perform due diligence on the lawful supply of genetic tests in Australia, before catching the next flight back to Seattle. He coordinated his schedule carefully so he would meet up with Sally just as she flew in from LAX.

'The day that I was to fly out to the US I felt sick to my stomach,' says Sally. 'Even though I was excited by the prospect of growing our family, the thought of leaving Massimo terrified me. My mother moved into our home with one of her best friends to care for him while we were away and we had timetabled a steady stream of visits from friends, family and carers to support her throughout the week. We even asked Leah, our family doctor, to stick her head in. Our next-door neighbour, Jenna, was a nurse, so she was enlisted to pop in every night to give Massimo his medication, and our close friend and family accountant had our wills along with detailed instructions for how Massimo was to be cared for in the event that anything was to happen to us.'

By the time Sally boarded the plane she was a bundle of nerves. Wanting to be in the best possible health for the upcoming pregnancy, she avoided alcohol, already worried that her highly stressed state was creating a less than ideal environment for her future baby. She thumbed through magazines and books, not really taking anything in.

They had decided to keep the whole donor IVF process to themselves for now, so Stephen created an elaborate cover story that their trip to the United States was for advanced genetic tests, which required fresh blood, semen and saliva samples they couldn't send from Australia. If Sally were to fall pregnant, they would keep the news a secret for as long as possible. The couple had enough to worry about without the distraction of countless opinions on proceeding with IVF, let alone donor conception.

'Stephen told the story of our US trip with such confidence and filled it with so much genetic jargon that everyone became overwhelmed and tuned out within thirty seconds,' says Sally. 'Only a geneticist would have been able to challenge him towards the end, and then only on the basis of cost estimates rather than the science.'

As she hadn't told anyone what they had been going through over the previous eight weeks, Sally was ready to burst. She ended up dumping her whole story on the man seated next to her on the plane, who couldn't have been any older than twenty-five. 'Not sure what to say, he ordered drink after drink, all the while listening to me recount the events of our lives that had led to me being on this flight.'

In the United States, the donor had been given a trigger shot of hormones three days earlier to start producing eggs; a batch of twenty had been harvested, of which thirteen were successfully fertilised with Stephen's sperm. Sally and Stephen met with the reproductive specialist at Seattle Reproductive Medicine to discuss the number of embryos they would have transferred.

'Once again, Stephen and I, leaving no option unanalysed, had already debated this very topic vigorously prior to this discussion,' says Sally. 'We had decided we would transfer two embryos. Our goal was to maximise the chance of success. If we ended up with twins as a consequence then that would be great – we would just brace ourselves until we got through the first few years of the storm. At this stage Massimo's condition had yet to stabilise so we still felt as though we were racing against the clock.'

The fertility specialist soon put a massive kink in their perfectly laid plans. She strongly discouraged the transfer of more than one embryo, warning them of the higher risk of birth defects – the very issue that they were trying to avoid.

Alarmed, Sally was ready to heed her advice. Stephen, on the other hand, was not. He questioned the doctor about the options available for prenatal testing, and she went through the various screening tests that could be carried out during the pregnancy. The most accurate procedures, such as Chorionic Villus Sampling – where a small sample is taken from the placenta with a fine needle passed through the abdomen at around ten weeks – can exclude genetic conditions such as Down Syndrome. However, these procedures carry with them an associated risk of 1 per cent, and could also result in a premature end to the pregnancy. Sally was very uncomfortable with the prospect of these tests. She left the consultation despondent and confused.

They took a cab back into town and grabbed some lunch at a busy Italian restaurant in downtown Seattle. Stephen was heading back to Melbourne the same afternoon so he could be with Massimo, leaving Sally alone for the procedure which would take place thirty-six hours later. The final decision rested with her. They shared a pasta marinara, discussing how many embryos they should have transferred.

'Everything had been so meticulously planned up to this point and now I was starting to feel uncertain. But Stephen was committed to the original plan we had in place – we would transfer two embryos.'

'I am not afraid of risk, not because I enjoy taking it, but because I am determined to come up with strategies to help me accept it,' says Stephen. 'Risk-based decision-making is intended to reduce the likelihood or consequence of a potential future event. It is not intended to reduce risk to zero, simply to a level that one can accept. We were only going to have one shot at a fresh embryo transfer before they were frozen. I'd researched IVF figures and there was a statistically significant drop in the success rate between fresh transfers and frozen transfers for Sally's age group. We had put in all this work and needed to make a decision to maximise the chances of success first time around. It was a simple decision based on probability – two fresh embryos.'

Still confused and scared, Sally wanted to talk about this

further, but Stephen had to get his flight, and in his mind there was absolutely nothing to discuss. 'He told me, in no uncertain terms, that his position was clear. We understood the risks and it was what we had agreed before boarding our flights to the United States. He wasn't going to be there for the transfer and if I wanted to change course I would be responsible for the outcome. I grew extremely frustrated at his dogmatic stance. We'd been on this journey together from the outset and now, at the most critical point, we were parting ways.'

Stephen's frustration with Sally's indecision mounted through the course of lunch. She couldn't understand why he could not indulge her in an analysis of the pros and cons; in his mind they had made their decision and she was opening up a moot topic.

'I felt like it was a lose–lose situation. If I stuck to our plan, I risked a pregnancy that could result in birth defects. In the event that a severe problem was discovered in one of the babies early enough we could undergo a selective reduction – a procedure that seemed at odds with the life-creating process of IVF – and risk losing the entire pregnancy. On the other hand, I could go ahead with the transfer of a single embryo and significantly reduce our chances of getting pregnant, potentially resulting in the need for more IVF cycles. That would mean a sibling for Massimo was even further away and possibly would not happen during his lifetime.'

A few hours later, Stephen was airborne, travelling to Los Angeles to board his flight home.

'I was, quite literally, alone,' Sally says.

She mulled her options over and over again as she wandered through the streets of Seattle the next day. She had organised to meet Melinda in person the night before the transfer, and was a bundle of nerves waiting for her in Starbucks. She had some gifts, which seemed so small and pathetic given the gift that Melinda was giving them.

'I recognised her immediately from the photos when she walked in. She wore a skirt and black coat, with high heels. She was striking, with her long, dark hair pulled off her face into a high ponytail. She picked me out immediately – I must have been that obvious, sitting there shaking like a leaf.'

The two women, strangers until that moment, chatted freely about the whole process. Melinda was still recovering from the egg collection and feeling the side effects of all of the medication she had been required to take. Even though there was a financial consideration, Sally, with her deep-seated compassion for others, couldn't help but feel bad.

'I didn't want her to suffer for helping us.'

Melinda reached out and took Sally's hand, reiterating that she had intended to remove herself from the donor register but had decided not to when she heard Massimo's story. Sally shared her anxieties about the transfer the next day but avoided mentioning her dilemma as she didn't want to burden Melinda. The two chatted about how Massimo was doing. Melinda told Sally a bit about her boyfriend and mentioned that her mother had been right by her side all along. It comforted Sally to be reassured Melinda hadn't had to go through the whole process alone.

'It was quite surreal,' says Sally, reflecting on the experience. 'Here was a complete stranger who, because of some amazing scientific advancements that have made egg donation possible, and through her own kindness, had just become part of the fabric of our life. I was feeling overwhelmed by the sheer enormity of the situation. I didn't know how to thank her enough. What I couldn't quite get across in words, I tried through a hand squeeze and hug. I don't think either of us expected to click the way we did, but it was as if we had known each other for years. Before I knew it Melinda had to leave and I was alone again with my thoughts. I headed back to the hotel to rest up for what lay ahead.'

The next morning, Sally went back to Seattle Reproductive Medicine for the egg transfer. She was escorted from the warm and bustling main reception area to a quieter spot down the hall where the procedure would take place. She was instructed to change into a gown and lie down on the treatment table in a small dark room. She had drunk several glasses of water as the procedure was to be guided by ultrasound, so she was at bursting point by the time things got underway.

'The on-call fertility specialist came in to introduce himself and was followed by the embryologist, who had come in to show me the embryo they had selected for the transfer. She gave me a photo of an embryo in a dish and told me that it was of excellent quality – in her opinion one of the best she had seen.'

Sally had reluctantly decided to go along with Stephen's wishes to transfer two embryos, but was dissuaded yet again by the team's recommendation not to. Wrought with indecision, she asked to call Stephen back in Melbourne. The fertility specialist spoke to him, but he reiterated that it was to be his wife's choice. Both the doctor and embryologist appeared relieved when Sally went with their advice, and within a few minutes one embryo was implanted. They left her alone to change and go to the bathroom, and when she returned the room was empty. No one was in the reception area either. She sat for a while wondering what to do and eventually left, feeling a little deflated.

'I'm not sure what I'd expected, but it was hard to believe that a life might have been created as a result of this cold and impersonal process. I left the clinic and hailed a cab, clutching the picture of my little embryo, our future baby. I flew back to Melbourne later that night.'

In between Christmas and New Year, Sally had a pregnancy test. The next day they paced around the house, hovering around the fax machine as they waited for the results. It came through mid-afternoon and was negative.

'I wasn't pregnant. After all that, the transfer had failed. It was my fault – I'd made the wrong decision. I've never seen Stephen look more disappointed. He didn't say anything and just walked out of the room. Distraught, I went straight to our bedroom. I lay on my bed, sobbing. And I had no one to turn to because we had kept the whole thing secret – no one I could ring, no girlfriend I could go and talk to, no shoulder to cry on.'

They will never know if transferring two embryos would have worked, or if the stress and the flight had affected Sally. But they did know they weren't going to make the same mistake again. They needed to take whatever actions were necessary to increase their chances.

Towards the end of 2009, Rick Leventer had made a further attempt to rule out any remaining rare genetic conditions. From mid-October to November, vials of Massimo's DNA were sent off to the United States and Italy for testing. Sally and Stephen were told that the timeframe for any answers would likely be several months, at best.

After a few weeks, Stephen received notification that one of the specimens had been held up in Italy.

'I couldn't believe it. Here was my son fading away before my eyes, and this precious DNA sample that could hold the key to a diagnosis couldn't get through Italian Customs and Quarantine due to some missing paperwork. No one could tell us what was required. To the FedEx call centre staff in the Philippines we were just another one of their ten million daily shipments. Each call or email enquiry was going to and fro between three countries, across three time zones in three different languages, and it was taking twenty-four hours to get a response. We were working on different timescales of what constituted urgent. I've been able to deliver Eyre BioBotanics orders to customers at Bagram Airbase in Afghanistan within seventy-two hours between mortar attacks by Taliban insurgents, but we couldn't get a humble medical specimen to a lab in Italy.'

Stephen emailed a contact at the Australian Trade Commission in Milan to ask for help pushing things through. He had worked closely with her previously to get Eyre BioBotanics distribution into Europe. She liaised with the head of the laboratory responsible for overseeing the test in Italy. There was a problem with the hygiene certificate, or rather the lack of one. It would only cost 20 Euros to issue, but FedEx didn't know who to charge. Finally, fifteen days after leaving Melbourne, the DNA sample arrived at the Giannina Gaslini Institute in Genoa.

Stephen was hugely relieved the sample had got through, but the stress was starting to take a toll on him. By mid-January 2010 Stephen was both mentally and physically broken.

'We'd just had our first Christmas together with Massimo since the devastating news of his condition, and thought it may well be the last. The initial IVF had failed and there was still tension in the house after our disagreement in Seattle. We'd missed our first opportunity and there was absolutely no way we weren't going to attempt a second transfer within four weeks. All this work was for Massimo and his siblings to meet, and the thought of him passing away while Sally was pregnant was sickening. Our plans to extend the house for Massimo and complete construction before having more children were falling behind schedule. The genetic tests from Italy were still in limbo and my mother was just about to start on a clinical trial for her advancing Alzheimer's disease. The world was spinning out of control.'

Meanwhile, Stephen was forced to step even further back from business commitments to focus on Massimo's diagnosis, as well as provide ever-increasing support to his ageing parents who were no longer able to take care of their own financial, legal and medical wellbeing.

'I was being slammed from every side. It seemed that every day, within minutes of waking, there was always another crisis I had to deal with. If ever there was a reason to have more than one child in a family, this was it. Being an only child meant I had to take on responsibility for everyone, which was personally and professionally crippling.'

Stephen had gone from being a relatively fit and healthy guy with a positive outlook and a growing start-up business, to someone under extreme stress 24/7.

'I packed on almost 15 kilos in the space of only six months and was leaning on a bottle of red every night to counteract the dozen coffees I was downing during the day – it was a vicious cycle of liquid stimulants and sedatives. Coupled with the fact I hadn't slept properly in six months and was eating junk at my desk just to survive, my body was starting to fail and I was regularly feeling faint when standing. On one occasion I collapsed while I was walking down the hall and thought I was about to die. It was a recipe for falling into depression and I knew I had to break the cycle, but I just didn't have five minutes to press pause and gather my thoughts. I wasn't going to be any use to Massimo if I got sick or had a heart attack.

I needed to commit to an epic physical challenge that was going to keep me in check for a long time and give me some mental respite, not something I could achieve with only partial focus. In the back of my mind I had thought about a marathon and mentioned it to Sally in passing a couple of times. But I was a rugby front row, not a runner, and at that point in time I couldn't run 50 metres without being out of breath.'

Stephen's birthday was on 19 January and Sally surprised him with what he now thinks was possibly the most important present of his life. It was a card with a Melbourne Marathon logo and picture of Massimo, and in it Sally had written, 'Brian Rabinowitz is expecting to see you at the gym tomorrow morning at 11 am. You are going to run a marathon and he will be your coach. See you at the finish line.' Before Massimo became ill, Stephen had attended Brian's legendary spin classes at 5.45 on Wednesday mornings.

'Brian is a consummate professional who commands respect within minutes of meeting him. If anyone was going to get my broad backside to run 42 kilometres, it was Brian. I explained everything that had happened to us over the previous six months and suffice to say he was shocked. Before training could start, I needed an all-clear from a doctor. I requested cardiac testing because I'd felt an irregular heartbeat on occasion, probably from all that caffeine, as well as the stress. On a VO2 max treadmill test I had to run until I was exhausted, which didn't take long in my case. The entire program would be based on graded heart rate training zones and over time we would work to build up my fitness. The first program involved me running for five minutes then winding down to an easy walk, but my heart was already pounding at 180 even before I got to the end of our street.'

Sally decided that another way to help Stephen get his health back on track was for her to return to work and help ease the financial burden.

'This was a huge relief, because it freed me to focus more on the diagnosis. Stepping back from a business I had worked so hard to build from scratch and watch it stagnate was difficult, but Massimo's and my health were priorities. I had built it once, and I would build it up again down the track.'

'Stephen and I share many similar values when it comes to working. If you want something you need to earn it. As the eldest daughter of hard-working migrants, I guess it was encoded in my DNA. Both my parents migrated to Australia straight after finishing high school, forgoing the opportunity to attend university. Instead, my father opted to travel to a foreign country on his own to forge the way for the rest of his family.'

Both Stephen and Sally feel lucky to have grown up with parents who worked hard to secure their children's futures.

'We obviously want to do the same for our children,' says Stephen. 'With the added degree of uncertainty around what lies ahead for Massimo, this is crucial. Working is not just about taking care of the here and now; it is about the future, ensuring we leave Massimo everything that he needs to be cared for, and cared for well. Not knowing what is in store for him and how long he might live, we need to plan for every possible permutation and combination that life throws at us.'

The one constant that has supported Sally's ability to work since Massimo was born has been her mother. While she hasn't always been the primary carer – down the track they also had carers, nannies and volunteers – Sally's mother has been very generous with her time.

'She accommodates our needs without question. When I first thought about returning to work after Massimo was diagnosed, she sat me down and explained that she was available 100 per cent to support us. She knew that while Massimo was still small he would be easier to care for. As he grew older and heavier, she might not be physically able to help as much.'

The next step in trying to have another child would involve either Sally going back to the United States for another transfer, or the embryos being brought to Australia. They decided to pursue the second option early in the New Year, but there was a hitch – legislation barred them from bringing frozen embryos that had been paid for into their home state of Victoria. Their local IVF specialist suggested that if they were able to arrange delivery of the embryos to Brisbane, where the use of paid eggs was permitted, he would refer them to a colleague at the Queensland Fertility Group to carry out the transfer.

'They wanted to transport them across all at once. Seattle Reproductive Medicine typically won't split batches of embryos,' says Stephen. 'You can be sure, though, I wasn't going to literally put all our eggs in one basket.'

He begged them to transport only half of the remaining embryos, posing all sorts of possibly drastic scenarios such as the transport vessel failing or the plane crashing. Finally they capitulated. Stephen and Sally had to pay $4000 for a private courier, who transported four out of their nine remaining frozen embryos across in his carry-on luggage.

With half of their embryos safely in Brisbane, Sally once more started the process of readying herself for the next transfer. She was able to artificially induce her cycle with the use of drugs and visited her local IVF clinic every couple of days for an ultrasound to determine if she was ready. She flew up to Brisbane in early February for the transfer, meeting the specialist on the morning of the procedure. Following the short consult she travelled from his rooms to the day centre where the procedure would take place.

'The bright and airy room was staffed with warm and caring nurses. I was asked to change into a gown and a fluffy terry towelling robe and take a seat in the lounge until the doctor was ready for me. A short while later I was shown into the treatment room. I was asked to get up on the bed and place my legs up in steel stirrups, leaving me exposed to the doctor who was still waiting for the embryologist to arrive with the two embryos they were planning to transfer. After what felt like forever she finally bounced into the room, declaring that the embryos looked so good they were almost ready to be checked into the childcare centre downstairs.'

The doctor swiftly implanted them. A few short minutes later, Sally was bundled back up in her robe and guided back into the lounge for a rest before being sent off.

'I was offered cheese and crackers and a brandy! What a difference to my first experience. When I was dismissed I headed back to the hotel and rested before my flight home. After our first disappointment I wasn't taking any chances.'

A few days prior to the blood test to check her HCG, or pregnancy hormone levels, Sally was feeling quietly confident that the second round of IVF would be successful. Feeling impatient, she bought a home pregnancy test to see if she could get an early reading. A pregnancy so early in the cycle would typically not have registered on a kit bought at the local pharmacy, but she decided to give it a go in any case.

'It was positive! We were pregnant!'

Sally cleaned the test and placed it on Stephen's desk, waiting for him to find it.

'My reaction was subdued. I was pleased, but more than that I felt a huge sense of relief. It felt like a vital project milestone had been achieved rather than a truly exciting moment. I remember being over the moon when finding out Sally was pregnant with Massimo. It wasn't the same this time; the whole process had been so clinical.

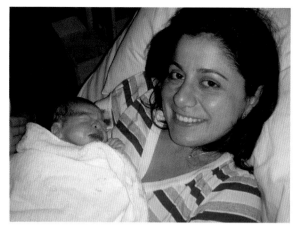

Massimo joins our world, 22 July 2008.

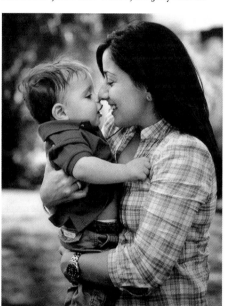

The first sign that something wasn't quite right: Massimo's toes starting to curl.

Creating memories: Massimo with Sally, September 2009.

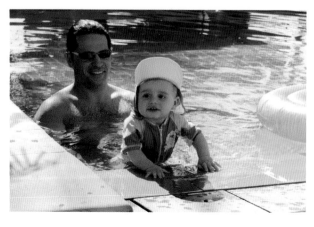

The first family holiday at Westin Denarau Resort in Fiji, June 2009.

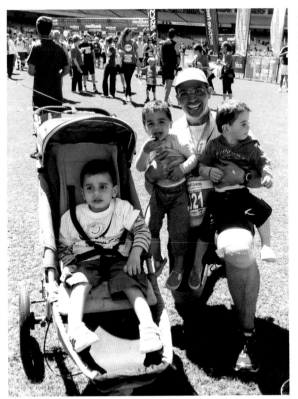

Stephen with Massimo, Marco and Leonardo at the MCG after crossing the finish line of his first marathon, October 2012.

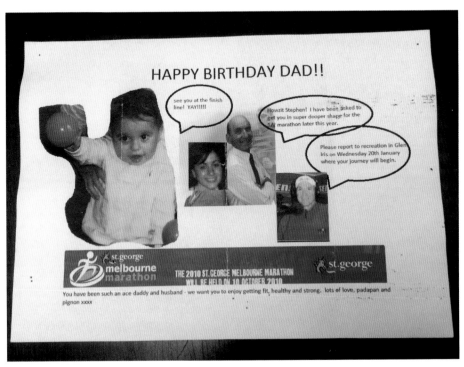

The original birthday invitation Sally made for Stephen.

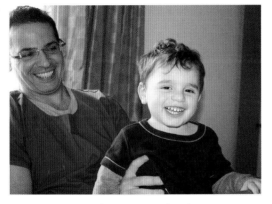

Massimo visiting his new twin brothers, Frances Perry Hospital, Melbourne, September 2010.

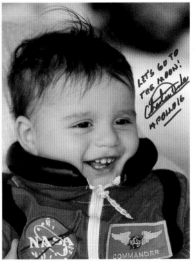

'Let's go to the moon!' Inspiration from astronaut Charles 'Charlie' Duke, CAPCOM Apollo 11 and Lunar Module Pilot Apollo 16. Duke signed copies of this photograph for all of the local members of the Mission Massimo Scientific Crew who were involved in achieving the diagnosis.

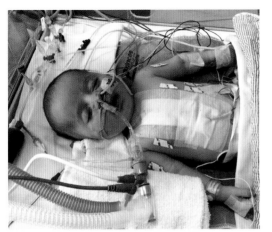

Leonardo in ICU at the Royal Children's Hospital following cardiac surgery to perform a VSD closure, December 2010.

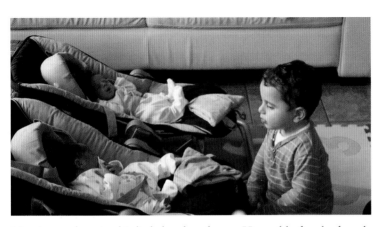

Massimo welcoming his little brothers home. He could often be found sitting at the end of their bouncers watching them intently.

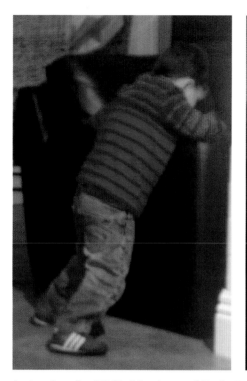
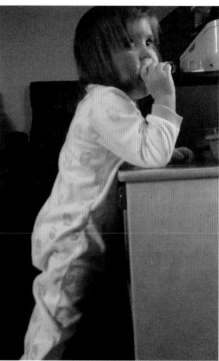

A giant leap for HBSL: Massimo and Emily Rose both pull to a standing position for the first time following their experimental corticosteroid infusions.

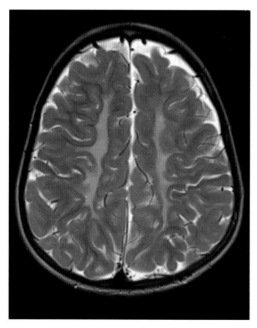

Massimo's MRI, October 2014, showing a slight improvement from his previous imaging.

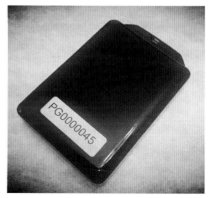

The hard drive with Massimo's whole genome delivered from Illumina.

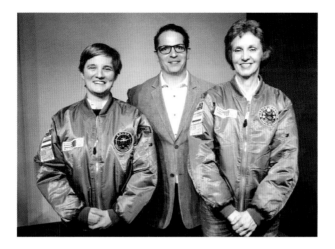

Stephen with Dr Adeline Vanderver and Professor Marjo van der Knaap at the Global Leukodystrophy Initiative meeting in Washington DC, January 2015.

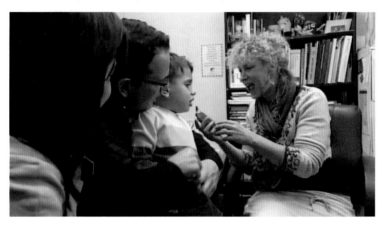

Massimo paying Dr Leah Kaminsky a visit in the clinic.

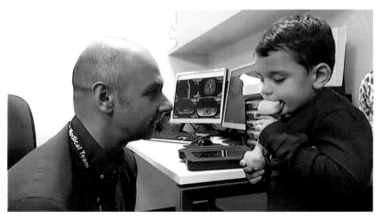

Massimo with Dr Rick Leventer during a routine visit at the Royal Children's Hospital in Melbourne.

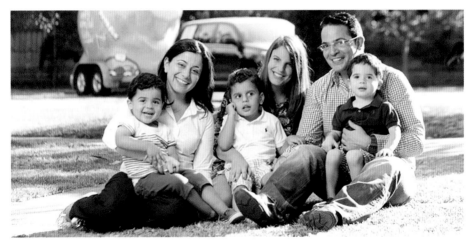

The Damianis with carer Jo Hendler – now Massimo's godmother and part of the family.

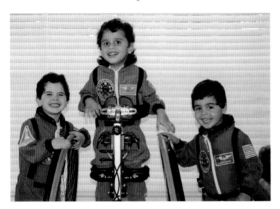

Team Massimo! Junior commanders providing inspiration to the Mission Massimo Running Crew at the first major Mission Massimo Foundation fundraiser.

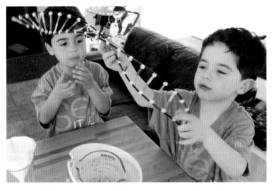

'We want to help Dr Ryan make special medicine when we grow up.' Marco and Leonardo getting a head start extracting DNA from kiwifruit with a home DNA kit.

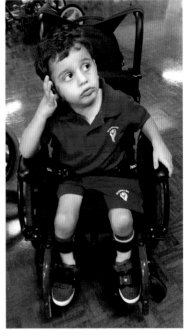

Defying the odds: Massimo on his first day of school, January 2014.

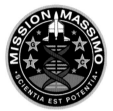 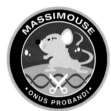 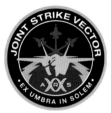 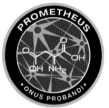

Each Mission Massimo Foundation project has its own patch recognising the efforts of all the teams involved.

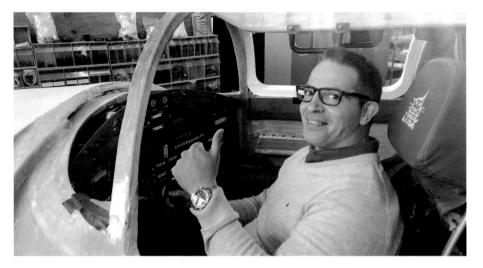

We are sending someone into space! Stephen has the opportunity to sit in the spacecraft at XCOR headquarters.

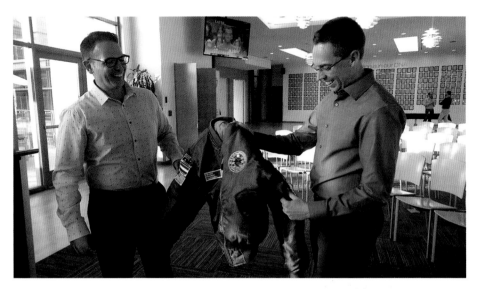

Stephen presents Ryan Taft with a Mission Massimo crew jacket emblazoned with the mission badges during a visit to Illumina, November 2014.

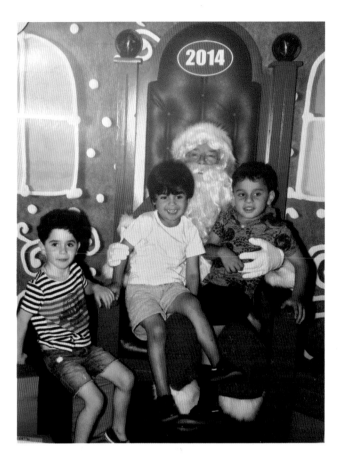

Marco, Massimo and Leonardo visit Santa, Christmas 2014. A happy time once again.

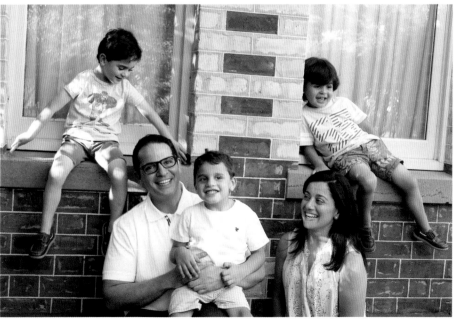

Looking forward to 2015.

I was reading a *Nature Genetics* paper at the time and just kept reading.'

A couple of days later the result was confirmed with a blood test. It was then, when the reality had sunk in, that Stephen allowed himself to feel a little excited. They visited their specialist at Melbourne IVF who did an early ultrasound, confirming the presence of two foetuses.

'We were having twins!' Sally was cautiously optimistic. 'He did warn us that one of the foetuses looked a little small and there was a chance it may not survive. We were advised it might be wiser not to tell anyone yet. Now, officially pregnant, he referred us to a high-risk obstetrician who would look after us from this point on. Nothing was going to be left to chance.'

Chapter 8

THE MASTER PLAN

'Meanwhile, alongside the excitement of twin boys growing inside Sally, we were watching our little son Massimo dying,' says Stephen.

In late January of 2010, Massimo had another MRI scan. The local radiologist reported that all was stable and largely unchanged. The MR imaging remained consistent with hypomyelination – an abnormally small amount of myelin in the brain.

Four months had passed when they finally received the remaining results from Italy excluding Hypomyelination with Congenital Cataract, with no abnormalities found in the FAM126A gene. Professor Marjo van der Knaap also reviewed Massimo's new MR imaging and sent her report in early May of 2010. Contrary to the local report, she noted significant changes, and put forward the possible grim diagnosis of Vanishing White Matter Disease, a condition where myelin is formed normally but after a period starts to break down and disintegrate (demyelination). Although Massimo's clinical presentation didn't really fit this diagnosis, she felt he could be in the very early stages of the disease.

'We had also sent his MR imaging from July 2009 to Kennedy Krieger in the United States for a second opinion. They came back suggesting delayed myelination rather than hypomyelination, as well as involvement of grey matter of the brain, a different type of tissue. The grey matter of the brain is responsible for muscle control, hearing, memory, emotions, speech and decision-making, whereas white matter contains the wiring to connect it all together.'

What was clear was significant disparity in the highly specialised interpretation of Massimo's MR imaging. Three different expert opinions didn't fill Stephen and Sally with confidence they would be able to reach a diagnosis in a meaningful timeframe for Massimo.

'We were using MR imaging of his brain to guide the diagnosis. Working on the basis of changes occurring over six- to twelve-month intervals, together with historical information about the nature and timing of symptoms, was less than ideal. We were watching and waiting for Massimo to get worse to provide us with direction for a diagnosis. Documenting the life, and ultimately death, of our son to achieve what might be a post-mortem diagnosis seemed to be a blunt approach.'

If they were going to save Massimo they needed a way to predict and prevent a future outcome. Stephen figured it made sense to search all of Massimo's genes in parallel to identify the cause. If the disease was presumed to be genetic and 50 per cent of these disorders remain undiagnosed, then surely the answer lay in the data of Massimo's DNA?

Stephen became more and more convinced that the idea of simultaneously analysing all of the genes in Massimo's genome was the way forward – the mapping of his entire DNA make-up, in order to identify the faulty gene.

'At that time I didn't understand the difference between clinical medicine and research. I wasn't a medico – naively, I thought it was just a case of "you wear a white coat, do whatever it takes". That's what always happened in *Grey's Anatomy*. You never saw McDreamy throw his hands up in the air and say, "You need to talk to the research guy." He'd just walk over to Joe's Bar, right across from Seattle Grace Hospital, knock down a couple of Scotches, then arrive back at work the following morning, with his signature McDreamy smile and perfect hair, having discovered the cure for spinal cancer. I soon realised that was all Hollywood.'

In early 2010, when Sally and Stephen first met Massimo's physiotherapist from Specialist Children's Services their main objective was to keep Massimo as comfortable as possible. Early on the sessions involved some gentle massage or a few suggestions on seating positions. One afternoon, however, as Sally sat on the play mat with Massimo in her lap as usual, the physiotherapist asked her to put him on the floor.

'I baulked at this suggestion. Ever since Massimo started to regress he spent most of his time either seated in my lap, being carried around on my hip, or strapped into a piece of equipment. It felt cruel to leave him lying alone, not being able to do anything, so I avoided it. I was always hovering around as his personal safety net. But the physio seemed convinced we were going to get him rolling again. Although I was sceptical, I agreed to give it a try. It didn't happen straight away, but over the course of a month he slowly rolled from his back to his side. Soon after that he managed to roll onto his tummy, and not long after followed with a full roll. Massimo was on the move again!'

Over the first half of 2010 Massimo's condition appeared to stabilise and he actually regained some lost skills. This was unusual for a child with Leukodystrophy. Stephen and Sally reached a point where all of the available literature on Leukodystrophies that described possible outcomes was quickly becoming irrelevant to Massimo. They found it staggering to see him crawling again and a tremendous relief. He was writing his own story.

In an effort to help Massimo learn to communicate, Sally showed him pictures of common objects such as water, food and his beloved Wiggles. To her surprise, he pointed to the ones he wanted.

'It was typically the picture of the colourful Wiggles

logo he wanted most, but nonetheless we had found a way for Massimo to indicate his needs beyond the use of tears and screams of frustration.'

Spurred by this progress, Sally spent an entire day taking photos of every object in the house Massimo might ever want, including all of his toys and many of his books, painstakingly laminating each photograph to fill an entire box.

'We were slowly starting to draw Massimo out of the shell that he had retreated into following the onset of his illness. It's hard to know why he was starting to develop again. Stephen and I often wonder if it was the intensity of all those hospital visits, the prodding and poking, the endless agonising procedures and the sheer terror that went along with it that had sent him hurtling backwards until then. Maybe in some way he felt scared because of the rapid onset and pace of his deterioration, reflected in the anxiety that must have showed on our faces. It was most likely a combination of factors, but one thing is for sure, as soon as the rate of hospital visits slowed down, so too did the pace of Massimo's regression.'

Once the pregnancy with the twins was confirmed, Stephen and Sally booked a brief family holiday to the Gold Coast while the house was being modified to accommodate Massimo's disabilities. They decided to take Massimo to the theme parks in an attempt to regain some sense of normality in their lives. They planned for Massimo to visit Wiggles World first, and then go on to Wet'n'Wild and Sea World. They wanted to spend time away as a family and make some fun-filled memories together. For the most part they felt like any other family, particularly when the three of them sat at breakfast. Massimo was still small enough to fit into a highchair, and to all intents and purposes looked like any other toddler, except for the spasticity in his legs that meant he couldn't really sit up properly.

'One morning we were having breakfast at our usual table,' says Stephen. 'Another family walked past and sat next to us. It was Michael Schumacher. Being a Formula 1 fan I recognised him immediately and gave him a knowing nod and smile. Massimo was starting to get a little restless and dropped his Wiggles Big Red Car on the floor. Michael picked it up, said hello and gave it back to him. I jokingly told Massimo that this man used to drive a really fast Big Red Car. Michael laughed.'

Later that day they all played in the pool. Massimo shrieked in delight as he splashed around, with Stephen treading water beside him. 'Touch my nose!' Stephen said, grinning, and Massimo reached out to grab him. It was a game he would soon not be able to play any more.

'We had to be creative and make up some new types of normal,' says Sally. 'Thanks to my smallish frame, I managed to squeeze myself into the little seats on the theme-park rides designed for children. This meant I could prop Massimo up on my lap because he wasn't able to sit up on his own. Depending on the ride, this often came with a fair amount of begging the attendant to let me on. Once

I explained our predicament they usually let us, but there were times we were turned away, for reasons of safety or some other policy. It gave us an insight into a strange new world, where not everything would be instantly accessible.'

In some ways, Sally feels this trip, as well as Massimo's condition stabilising, began to set the tone for the new type of life they were determined to have.

'We were going to treat Massimo like any other child. We would go to the park because that is what toddlers do, and I would climb up onto all of the equipment with him on my hip, go down all of the slides and swing for ages with Massimo on my lap. I just made it work. Most of the time the confused looks from the other parents didn't bother me, but sometimes they would break through the thin veneer of composure I had built around myself and I would cry as I walked Massimo back home in the stroller.'

Around this time, Stephen and Sally feel there was an unconscious transition from caring for what they thought was a dying child, to raising a child with severe special needs. Up until then, Massimo had been deteriorating in all ways. Stephen and Sally had been preparing themselves for the worst. After his symptoms started to plateau, the focus gradually shifted from grieving for their anticipated loss to fierce determination to help their son.

While they celebrated all the small gains that Massimo was making, everything was still layered with a tremendous sense of anxiety. They were deeply concerned that although he was stabilising, his development was far too slow.

'If we noticed any small change we'd analyse it to bits,' Sally says. 'When Massimo coughed or choked on a piece of food, I would go into a tailspin – was this a new sign that he was regressing? Would we need to take the next step that was often the case with these conditions and start considering tube feeding to avoid aspiration? Thankfully these episodes were few and far between.'

Illness can be like a foreign country to those blessed with good health. One of Sally's favourite poems is 'Welcome to Holland' by Emily Perl Kingsley. Written by the mother of a disabled child, it describes the disorientation and disbelief when 'there's a change in the flight plan' and a child you expected to be perfectly healthy becomes unwell, diverting you on a different journey. Kingsley likens it to having a plan to go to Italy: you read up all about it and work out your itinerary, but when your plane instead lands in Holland, you are stranded there, with no guidebook and unable to speak the language. Meanwhile, 'everyone you know is busy coming and going from Italy . . . and they're all bragging about what a wonderful time they had there'. The message at the end of the poem is that if you spend your life mourning that you didn't get to your intended destination, you will never notice the wonderful things about the country you are actually in.

Stephen and Sally weren't quite at the point of appreciating the tulips and windmills in Holland. For a start, as the reality of Massimo's illness began to sink in, Sally and Stephen felt a growing awareness of the unexpected gulf that was developing between themselves and some of their friends whose children were healthy.

'While our close friends were still there, things felt different,' says Sally. 'I was willing to give most things a go with Massimo in tow, but I had to accept that this didn't always work. We took Massimo to countless birthday parties in all manner of places, and sometimes he would have a wonderful time, but more often than not the crowded venues and the noise would result in sensory overload and we found ourselves rushing out the door to placate our distressed son. No one ever begrudged us, but when the next invitation arrived I would always feel conflicted: should I take Massimo along in case this was one of the times he enjoyed himself or keep him at home where I knew he would be happy and content? Keeping him at home felt like giving up so I would always give it a go, even if it meant our trips were really short and we had to endure looks of pity as we rushed out the door with a hysterical child, leaving our friends to explain to their confused children what was going on.

'After a while I started to realise that my friends were beginning to keep their personal issues from me because they felt I had too much to worry about or that their problems were trivial in comparison. I was hurt when I learned a close friend didn't share that she was having difficulty conceiving her second child. It wasn't malicious or intentional, but it created a divide that added to my sense of isolation.

'Play dates also took on a whole new direction. Most

children would be left to play freely with one another while the mums shared a coffee and a gossip, but I often had to hang out with the kids, propping Massimo up so he could play along with the other children and not miss out. I wouldn't have had it any other way – he was happy and the kids all loved it – but it made it hard to feel like one of the girls.

'We suddenly had no more dreams of Massimo speaking several languages, or winning sporting trophies. There would be no academic achievements, no musical prowess, no go-karting, rugby, swim squad,' says Sally. 'Not only would Massimo never develop any of these skills, he wasn't even going to walk independently. We would never see him toddle up the hallway or run around in the backyard with the dog. And he would never utter the words *mum* and *dad*. We were never going to get to our original destination of Italy.'

Award-winning writer Andrew Solomon writes in *Far from the Tree: Parents, Children and the Search for Identity* that for the parents of children with life-threatening conditions the dissonance between the child they wanted and the child they end up with can lead to profound tension in the dynamics of other relationships. 'Perhaps the most insidious stress is the social isolation that can ensue when friends retreat, or when parents withdraw from friends' incomprehension.'

'In the first few months following Massimo's dreadful MRI result, we were connected with a number of support groups offering to help us in some way,' says Sally. 'They would ask us what we needed and, to be honest, most of the time we had no idea. We simply didn't know what we should be asking for, or what would help with the situation that we were in. During one of these visits, a lady who introduced herself as Massimo's case manager offered to arrange some respite care through the local council for Massimo, to give us a break. I half-heartedly agreed, but really had no intention of handing my son over to a stranger, even for a few hours. A week later I received a call informing me that a lady named Jo would come over to our house on Friday morning to care for Massimo. I was told that if we liked her she could visit every week.'

Jo – or JoJo as the Damiani family call her – remembers when she was first asked about taking the shift with Massimo.

'I wasn't keen on the 8 am start, but I couldn't resist looking after a young baby. My boss at the time warned me not to get too attached, that they were expecting that Massimo may be in palliative care within a few months.'

'A quietly spoken young woman in her early twenties greeted me at the door on the Friday morning, introducing herself as Jo Hendler,' says Sally. 'I invited her in to meet Massimo before informing her that I would spend her three-hour shift with her, to help her get to know Massimo and understand his needs. She seemed a little taken aback. I am assuming most other parents seize the opportunity for a bit of quiet time and sanity, but she went along with what I was asking. I'm not sure what I was worried about: Massimo, despite being cautious of most people he came across, took to her immediately. An hour or so later Jo suggested that she could take Massimo for a walk to the park. "I'll come with you!" I immediately replied, jumping to my feet. Jo agreed and we spent a lovely morning at the park chatting and getting to know one another. When we returned home, I left her alone for the last half an hour to play with Massimo. While the two of them played, I walked into Stephen's study and declared, "I like this girl; she's a keeper."'

It was the first time Sally felt she might be able to share the care of Massimo with someone other than her mother.

'It was just beautiful watching the special bond that Jo and Massimo developed over the course of her weekly visits. She was gentle and intuitive, and seemed to be able to tap into that secret language that I have with Massimo, anticipating and meeting all of those unspoken needs he is unable to communicate. However, it's when she's pushing him to do his therapy that the true love she has for Massimo can be seen, because she knows it will be good for him in the long run. She will sit out a tantrum because she, like me, knows he eventually needs to learn that he will not get his way with everything just because he can scream loudly. She always lugs his huge communication book around and uses it religiously, even when Massimo does not appear to be paying attention. You know someone really cares for your child when they become just as excited about their small achievements as you do. Jo often sent a text to me whenever Massimo accomplished something, or even did something as mundane as sit through a whole book, or take a bite of a piece of fruit he wouldn't normally eat.

You don't get excited about things like that unless you are emotionally invested, unless you love someone. In some ways Jo has grown up with us as we have all adapted to the changing course of Massimo's illness. We joke about being her second parents, and in many ways Jo is the sister and daughter that I never had, all in one.'

Other than fitting under the loose umbrella term of Leuko-dystrophy, Stephen and Sally still had no idea what was wrong with Massimo. Vanishing White Matter – a brutal name for a disease if ever there was one – had been placed on the list of possible diagnoses, but testing the five genes associated with it was going to cost US$5000 at Baylor University in Texas. Unfortunately, none of the limited public funding for genetic testing was made available. It was due to a policy of only funding external genetic testing if there was a prenatal counselling or diagnosis question, where the outcome of the testing would affect immediate family-planning decisions or provide a specific treatment.

'Paradoxically, because we had proceeded with a donor pregnancy and there was no risk to the twins,' says Stephen, 'we would receive no further financial support through the public system for genetic testing. And our private health insurance didn't cover it. From this point on, we were on our own financially for further genetic testing to diagnose Massimo. The medical team was hamstrung by the perennial and difficult problem of limited government funding and resources. At the time it was a real blow. Effectively, the financial responsibility, if we wanted to pursue a diagnosis, had been passed to us. Looking back, it may have been a blessing in disguise.'

Stephen remembers saying in one meeting with Rick, 'It's just a broken gene, it's just statistics, it's just data. We need everyone to focus on the science and let us worry about the money. Whatever the cost, we'll find a way.'

'Effectively,' says Stephen, 'this also meant that we took over control of driving the pace of the diagnosis to a far greater degree, but we would now become the financial bottleneck. We were also now personally accountable to Massimo for achieving the diagnosis.'

This was Massimo's own moon-shot project, and Stephen had just become the Mission Massimo Flight Director.

'By early 2010 the cost of sequencing a genome had come down to a not insignificant but somewhat more affordable US$45,000. It was no longer an abstract figure in the tens of millions.'

Analysing the child and parents' genomes in parallel all seemed pretty straightforward in theory. In practice, however, Stephen soon found out that this wasn't being done on a regular basis and analysing the data for only one affected child – rather than a whole cohort – wasn't going to be easy. If a gene of interest was found, it would always be difficult to prove a diagnosis with a sample of only one patient.

'Not easy,' he says. 'But not impossible!'

Stephen knew that a sequential gene-by-gene approach was going to take too long, and so in mid-May 2010 he picked up the phone and dialled the number of a biotechnology company in San Diego called Illumina. Their mission statement is: 'To advance human health by unlocking the power of the genome.'

Stephen has the exact date and time of that call captured in his records – 18/5/2010 at 9.23 am Australian EST.

'Hello, I'm calling from Melbourne, Australia, and I'd like some more information on ordering a whole genome,' Stephen said to the man on the other end of the phone.

'I'm sorry, sir, can you repeat that?'

'A whole genome. It's on your website.'

Pause.

'It is? Okay. I'm just going to put you on hold for a minute.'

A minute passed and the man came back on the line. 'I'll have to take down your details and have someone get back to you.'

A couple of days later Brett Kennedy, Illumina's representative in Melbourne, contacted Stephen, advising him that it was a very new service and had never been requested in Australia. He needed to confirm what the specimen requirements would be and check the logistics of ordering it through a clinician. The cost was indeed going to be approximately US$45,000 to have Massimo's whole genome mapped.

'Yes, it was a lot of money but we had no other option. This was our best and last chance at a diagnosis. We also had to be prepared to sequence our parental genomes next.

Science was finally doing the talking, but finance was doing the walking.'

On 3 June, Brett Kennedy forwarded an email from Illumina announcing that 'individuals with serious medical conditions for whom whole-genome sequencing could be of clinical value will only have to pay US$9500 to have their genome sequenced, if ordered through a research institute'.

'Any chance of a three for two discount?' Stephen asked, half-joking.

In the media release, Jay Flatley, the company's president and CEO said, 'So far, Illumina has sequenced the genomes of fourteen individuals through the service, including those of former Solexa CEO John West and his four-member family, two centenarians, one cancer patient, and an infant with a known genetic disease where the under-lying mutation is unknown.'

Because a test of this kind had never been ordered locally before, Stephen and Sally had to wait for Victorian Clinical Genetic Services, Murdoch Children's Research Institute and Illumina ethics approval. On 24 June 2010, a sample collection kit for the Illumina FastTrack Whole Genome Sequencing Services was shipped.

'I tracked it every step of the way from San Diego to Melbourne, and when I saw it held up in Sydney for Australian Customs and Quarantine inspections I was on the phone to FedEx in minutes. We weren't going to have another delay like in Italy. Nonetheless, it frustratingly still took several days to clear.'

Finally, on 13 July 2010 a small vial of Massimo's blood was collected at the Royal Children's Hospital and was airborne, on its way by the afternoon to Illumina in San Diego for DNA extraction and sequencing.

Stephen and Sally didn't always notice a change in Massimo's abilities, and so it was with some dismay that they received the news that a follow-up MRI scan and eye exam in August 2010 had confirmed that his condition was deteriorating. The most alarming piece of information was the confirmation of an abnormality in Massimo's eyes.

'The potential loss of sight was one of the most horrifying pieces of news we received following the shock of his initial diagnosis,' says Sally. 'Massimo's gorgeous, expressive eyes were one of his main methods of communication, always telling us when he wanted something, when he was happy or sad. He loved watching kids' TV shows, looking at picture story books and playing with his iPad.'

'There was always a question mark about this abnormality in his eyes,' adds Stephen, 'and his ophthalmologist, Dr James Elder, could never say for certain it was a cherry red spot, which was often seen in severe forms of Leukodystrophy such as Krabbe Disease. Rather, he would tell us something wasn't quite right. It was a finding a specialist might only see once in their entire career. After Massimo's MRI in August 2010, Dr Elder reviewed his eyes in recovery while he was still under general anaesthetic. "Unfortunately, I can say with absolute certainty what I am seeing is a cherry red spot." I felt physically sick hearing those words and thinking Massimo was going to lose his sight.'

Without a known genetic diagnosis, Massimo's course of treatment often involved a fair amount of trial and error. One of the trials included a drug often prescribed to patients with Parkinson's disease called L-DOPA. It seemed to have an immediate impact, as he started to support himself, sitting up on the floor on his knees in a 'W' position. While this position was not ideal for the development of his hips, and was frowned upon by his physiotherapist, it gave Massimo a little more independence.

'It meant that he was able to sit on his own, not on my lap, and play with a toy. It was a huge gain and we celebrated. More floor time meant that Massimo started to regain some skills, the most exciting being his ability to crawl around. It was a far cry from the cross-pattern crawling he did before the onset of his condition, but it meant he was able to move around by himself, a huge gain.'

The drug, however, interfered drastically with Massimo's sleep. It became harder and harder to get him down at night and he would often wake a few hours later, shrieking. Scared that if they stopped the drug he would regress again, Stephen and Sally put up with the sleeplessness.

'Each time Massimo woke,' says Sally, 'I rushed to his bedside to soothe him, often lifting him up for a cuddle. It became increasingly difficult to get him to go back to sleep and I often paced the hallway with Massimo draped over my swelling pregnant belly. I would walk up and down the hallway, wait for him to fall asleep and put him back into bed. Sometimes I managed to steal a few hours sleep and other times the minute his body hit the mattress his eyes would pop open and he would start screaming again. It got to the point where I would need to hold him for a good hour before I could place him back in bed. Later in my pregnancy Massimo would fall asleep on my shoulder while I sat on the couch, but eventually I couldn't get up without disturbing him. I would send a text message to Stephen who would get out of bed to help me. Thinking that the L-DOPA had been responsible for the gains, we endured this difficult routine for almost two months.'

By early September, they took Massimo off the new medication. The lack of sleep had negated any progress he had made in development and it was no use being able to crawl if he spent the day miserable from exhaustion. The good news was that he continued to be able to kneel up and slowly crawl around.

It was at this time that Sally had her thirty-four-week antenatal ultrasound.

'The growth of one of our twins had slowed down. They told us not to be alarmed, but we would need to have intensive monitoring and the twins would need to be delivered early.'

Stephen and Sally decided they would benefit from some help. The first carer to start was an older woman. They interviewed her the week prior to ensure she understood Massimo's high care needs.

'She sounded like Mary Poppins,' says Stephen, 'promising us she would get our house back in order, improve

Massimo's sleep patterns and let us rest and recover. On her first day, though, she arrived over an hour late and then had to leave early because one of her kids had forgotten their key to the house. Later that evening we received a call from the agency to say it wasn't going to work out with this carer and Massimo. We felt she thought our little boy was a freak. It was such a blow.'

Luckily, a new carer, Siobhan, joined the family to help out.

'She was in her mid-thirties and full of energy. Initially she started as a night nanny. Within days she got Massimo back into a regular sleeping pattern. Before long she earned the title of "super nanny". She spent a lot of time talking to Massimo, trying to keep him engaged and stimulated.'

A week before the scheduled caesarean, Sally had foetal monitoring, followed by a further scan.

'Looks like we'll be having some babies tomorrow,' their obstetrician told them, smiling broadly.

The follow-up scan confirmed that one of the twins had stopped growing. At thirty-six weeks it was safe to have the babies and give the smaller twin a greater opportunity to thrive. When Sally was pregnant with Massimo her waters had broken in the middle of the night, so it felt strange going to bed knowing that she was going to have her babies the next day. After a relaxed drive into the hospital the following afternoon, they were admitted to the maternity ward. Half an hour later, Sally was lying on a gurney outside the operating theatre, leafing through a magazine.

'Stephen and I were idly chatting to the anaesthetist while

my obstetrician, assisted by one of his colleagues and the nurse, prepared for the caesarean. I turned to the anaesthetist who had just given me an epidural injection and asked him whether I would feel the incision. "Nope," he replied casually, "they've already done it." I was surprised at the pace at which things were moving and, before I knew it, baby number one was delivered, swiftly followed by baby number two. One of the nurses presented the twins to me, before whisking both of them away for a more thorough examination. While the doctor stitched me up, he asked if we had chosen names for them. Stephen and I had already decided on Marco and Leonardo, but didn't know yet which baby was to receive which name. "Why don't you give the small one the big name," the doctor suggested, and that's how we named our baby boys.'

Soon after, Stephen followed the twins up to the special-care nursery where they were to stay initially, while Sally was wheeled out to the recovery area.

'It felt weird lying in the quiet room all on my own, while my babies were on a different floor of the hospital being attended to by strangers. But I took comfort in the fact that everything appeared to be fine when they were first checked by the paediatrician.'

Minutes after the birth of Sally and Stephen's twin boys, Stephen was in the car driving across town to the Alfred Hospital, where his father had been rushed by ambulance following a respiratory attack earlier that day. It felt to Stephen and Sally a little as if history was repeating itself because Massimo's birth had also been overshadowed by family illness – in that instance by the realisation that Stephen's mother was exhibiting the early signs of Alzheimer's disease.

'Sally and I never had a chance to simply enjoy our children without some sort of crisis in the background or around the corner, be it Massimo's Spina Bifida Occulta, single kidney and tethered cord, or my mother's progressive dementia and the inherent difficulties involved.'

Sally felt sad that Stephen had so little time to spend with his newborn boys as he raced nonstop between hospitals, and made sure Sally's mum had everything she needed to look after Massimo. Seeing the exhaustion on his face as he sat on the end of her bed after having spent another long day at the Alfred Hospital with his father, she wished he had a brother or sister with whom to share the growing burden of caring for his ageing parents.

Massimo came in with Sally's mother and his new carer, Siobhan, who would remain with the family for many years, to visit his new brothers. He seemed happy, but it was hard to know whether he understood what was going on. The twins were discharged from the special-care nursery to a regular ward once their feeding routines became established and the staff felt confident that they were thriving. Even the smaller twin, Leonardo, appeared to be doing fine.

'A couple of days later, Stephen and I bundled the twins into their new stroller and made our way down to the car park. As I strapped the twins into their car seats, I started to feel the same sense of anxiety that I had experienced with Massimo. No more safety net at the end of a buzzer. Our boys were coming home.'

The first night found Sally huddled in a corner of the study, holding one twin in each arm, trying not to wake Massimo, who had only just started to sleep through the night.

'It was exactly like Massimo's first night at home after he was born – I don't know if I was just exhausted, but I actually had to laugh at the whole situation, thinking here we go again!'

They were right back to sleepless nights once more. However, the twins injected more than a sense of normality into the house – they also helped balance the intense focus that Stephen and Sally had placed on Massimo. And Massimo appeared happier too, as though he sensed everyone was relaxed. With his newly found ability to kneel up, he often sat between the two bouncers, smiling at his brothers. It showed Stephen and Sally that Massimo was still connected to what was going on around him.

'During the twins' feeding time Massimo would have a real tantrum, demanding their bottles and sometimes crawling over to snatch one away. We had a jealous sibling on our hands and we couldn't have been happier. The first few weeks were a blur of nappies, swaddling, bottles, burping and pooping. Whenever Stephen or I felt so exhausted we could barely keep our eyes open, we would remind ourselves that this part was only short term and there was light at the end of the tunnel.'

Life soon threw Stephen and Sally another detour, and that light at the end of the tunnel faded again. Stephen had sensed from the outset that something was not quite right with Leonardo. He was always a lot slower to feed, always struggling to finish a bottle, unlike his twin, Marco, who guzzled with gusto. He looked pale, his breathing was shallow and his skin felt cold to touch.

'Stephen always picks things well before anyone else,' says Sally. 'He can see the lie of the land and I often jokingly call him our "futurologist". In this instance I was praying that just for once he was wrong.'

Sadly, Stephen and Sally have become somewhat accustomed to crisis. Soon after the twins were born, they went to Leah Kaminsky's clinic for their routine six-week baby check. Marco, the first twin, was a robust, healthy baby who passed his examination with flying colours. Leah was about to announce a long-awaited 'Everything seems to be okay!' when she noticed a slight squint in one of his eyes. 'How was I going to tell this lovely couple, who had gone to hell and back with their firstborn, that another one of their children may have a problem? I played it down, explaining that a misalignment of eye muscles is an extremely common finding in newborns, usually disappearing by the time the baby reaches four months old. Even so, I could see Stephen's face drop as I told them he would need to be monitored by an eye specialist for a while.'

Leah soon turned her attention to little Leo, the smaller

of the twins. 'Sally was seated beside my desk holding him in her arms and I noticed he looked extremely pale. She told me he had been struggling to feed, getting exhausted and falling asleep well before he finished a bottle. As I went through a crucial part of the examination ritual, listening carefully to Leo's tiny chest, my own heart skipped a beat as I heard an extra noise: a cardiac murmur echoing through the bell of my stethoscope. It was a whooshing sound, characteristic of a hole in the heart, a fault in the development of the septum or wall between the two main chambers or ventricles. It was more than likely Leo was going to need an urgent operation. I felt nauseated, my lips tingling, a lump forming in my throat. Breaking bad news to patients has never been my forte, but with Stephen and Sally it was excruciating. What more could possibly go wrong for this young couple?'

Stephen's eyes widened in disbelief when Leah told them about the heart murmur. 'We're jinxed.'

He looked as if he had been startled by the headlights of an oncoming road train which was about to flatten him.

An ultrasound and ECG the same day confirmed the diagnosis of a Ventricular Septal Defect, more commonly known as a VSD, or hole in the heart. By the time they met with the cardiac surgeon, Stephen had a million questions he wanted to ask, but he was lost for words when Dr Yves d'Udekem, a tall Belgian doctor who lists one of his hobbies as didgeridoo playing, entered the room.

'I couldn't believe it. I remembered him from that awful

day, sixteen months earlier, as we waited for Massimo to come out of recovery after his MRI scan. This was the same doctor who had strolled into the waiting room and spoken to the family seated beside us. He had just finished a ten-hour heart operation on their child. I could hardly believe now it was our turn for Dr d'Udekem to be Leo's surgeon.'

Initially, Sally was quite rattled by the news and quietly wept while the specialist explained Leonardo's results.

'I wondered why this was happening to us, why we were once again in a position where the life of one of our children was at risk. The difference between Leonardo and Massimo, though, was there was a known solution to Leonardo's problem with an extremely high success rate. Once the VSD – the hole in Leonardo's heart – was repaired, he would go on to live a normal life with no further complications.'

Early on the morning of the surgery, Sally and Stephen made the now routine drive across to the Royal Children's Hospital, only this time it wasn't Massimo in the back seat but Leonardo, breathing his small shallow breaths. Stephen couldn't help but notice the weird coincidence of the letters of their car registration – VSD. As they walked through the main foyer of the hospital to take the lift to admissions, Sally also did a double take. They had just walked past a nurse who was the spitting image of their egg donor. It felt almost as though Melinda was there, watching over little Leonardo. Sally wondered if Stephen had noticed. She bit her tongue, afraid he would think that she was going crazy.

'When the same nurse entered the waiting room an hour or so later calling out Leonardo's name, I started to quietly freak out,' says Sally.

The doppelgänger nurse took routine temperature and blood pressure measurements and soon left to attend to another matter.

Stephen and Sally suddenly looked at each other in bewilderment, with the same thing on the tip of their tongues.

'She looks exactly like Melinda!'

Sally's next-door neighbour, Jenna, sat beside her in the waiting room for hours while Leonardo was in surgery, taking it in shifts with Stephen. Although they had been warned at the pre-admission briefing that he would come out of the operation with wires and tubes attached to his body, Sally still shuddered at the sight of her little baby surrounded by beeping machines.

'We'd also been warned about potential complications, both major and minor, that could occur after heart surgery. Leonardo experienced most of these, earning him an extra few nights in the ICU, which in a perverse way offered me some comfort. I was feeling torn about having to divide my time between the three boys. Knowing Leonardo was safe in ICU with round-the-clock care eased the guilt I felt about leaving him in hospital overnight on his own, something I'd never done with Massimo.'

In the same way he researched Leukodystrophy so thoroughly, Stephen had spent hours weighing up the risks of Leonardo's surgery. One of the greatest potential problems was 'Atrioventricular Conduction Block', caused by misfiring of nerves between the chambers of the heart that may inadvertently be cut during the repair of the ventricular septal defect. This meant the patient would require a permanent pacemaker. When Stephen saw wires running from Leonardo's abdomen to an external pacemaker as soon as he was wheeled into ICU he became concerned. They were reassured, though, that the cardiac surgery went smoothly and not long after, Stephen sat quietly beside Leo's crib, relieved to see the pacemaker was not turned on.

'The other parents must have thought I was either one cool customer or completely deranged as I tapped away, writing emails on my iPad, while they were desperately worried about their children. For us, in the scheme of things, this cardiac surgery was nothing compared to what we'd been through with Massimo. There was a diagnosis and well-tried solution to the problem. Dr d'Udekem does this kind of procedure every day. He was the guy we wanted. Sure, there were risks, but there was absolutely nothing I could do to change the outcome.'

Ten days later they took their baby boy home, the hole in his heart now repaired. Subsequent follow-ups confirmed the success of his surgery and they began to see their little baby thrive, now able to eat without becoming short of breath and exhausted. These days Leonardo proudly lifts up his T-shirt, showing off his scar to anyone willing to take a look.

'It's my zipper,' he says.

The typical course of Leukodystrophies is relentless from onset to death. However, Massimo continued to regain lost skills, as well as to maintain those he had already acquired. This was highly unusual. He was also developing greater spasticity in his legs than his arms, a unique symptom that puzzled his clinicians. Stephen set up a Google Alert for this feature using key words that described the symptoms.

When an email had popped into his inbox with a link to a paper, detailing a disorder called Leukoencephalopathy with Brain stem and Spinal cord involvement and high Lactate (LBSL), caused by a mutation in the DARS2 gene with a marked difference between upper and lower limb spasticity, he was astonished. Incredibly, the primary author for the paper was none other than Professor Marjo van der Knaap from Amsterdam.

'LBSL sounded like a perfect fit,' says Stephen, 'but I think we all assumed surely it would have come up previously.'

A disc with Massimo's MRI scan was sent to Professor van der Knaap for review. Once again she noted changes in the MR imaging, and sure enough she raised the possible diagnosis of LBSL with near-identical spinal cord changes.

Massimo's genome was being sequenced and local genetic services agreed to also review the DARS2 gene, along with the five genes for Vanishing White Matter Disease. It gave Stephen and Sally some hope that at least they were creeping closer to a diagnosis. Massimo's genome data was made available in mid-October, and in early November, on day 472 of their journey, the news came back that no abnormalities were detected in any of these genes.

'We had ruled out every known type of Leukodystrophy and Massimo was now in the 50 per cent undiagnosed category,' says Stephen. 'I felt a little defeated, although part of me was immensely relieved. Had the test for Vanishing White Matter Disease come back as positive, we would have had a diagnosis for sure, but it also would have meant a tragic prognosis for Massimo.'

As 2010 was drawing to a close, Stephen received an unassuming black USB HDD labelled PG0000045. He assumed the nomenclature was short for Personal Genome #45. At the time he had no idea it was actually one of the first ever genomes run through the Illumina clinical lab.

'Somewhere in the gigabytes of genetic sequence data was the answer we were looking for, but it may as well have been the black obelisk from *2001: Space Odyssey*, as I certainly felt like one of the apes staring at it in bewilderment. We seemed to have reached a dead end.'

Chapter 9

WHEN WATER IS THICKER THAN BLOOD

In times of need we turn to those nearest to us, looking for support and understanding. Traditionally, family is the first to be there; the ones to offer both a practical and emotional buttress against the onslaught of life-threatening illness. Sadly, though, some of Sally's extended family backed away completely when Massimo became ill in 2009, and then again in 2011 when he had to have neurosurgery to release his tethered spinal cord. Stephen and Sally have learned through bitter experience that blood isn't necessarily thicker than water.

'I think they just weren't able to deal with his sickness,' says Sally. 'It seems that it was easier to make it go away by ignoring it. I was told that they did not visit Massimo because it would be too upsetting. They had all attended

Massimo's baptism six months before, joyfully celebrating him in good health, but were not around when he became ill.'

Care and concern sometimes comes from unexpected places. Sally tells the story of how their regular FedEx driver arrived one afternoon for the daily pick-up of Eyre BioBotanics. The courier had also been the one to send Massimo's MR imaging and the hard drive of his genome out into the world.

'Early in the piece, when things with Massimo were deteriorating rapidly, he asked for a photo of Massimo, explaining that his family had arranged a special prayer service for him at their church.' Stephen and Sally were touched by this, but Sally also felt sad that a stranger seemed more concerned with Massimo's plight than blood relatives. When she confided in a close relative that they had decided not to attend a wedding where these extended family members would be, she was shocked at the response:

'What will happen if there's ever a family tragedy? You will need them then.'

Sally didn't know how to respond. Recounting the story five years later, her hands still tremble and tears well up.

'We were dealing with a terminally ill child. Isn't that tragic enough?'

Stephen took a much firmer stance.

'If Massimo having a fatal disease was not seen as a family tragedy, then the message was loud and clear to me – he was not considered family.'

Living under this cloud was causing ongoing stress for both of them, distracting them from what should have been their focus – finding a diagnosis for Massimo while providing him with the best quality of life possible.

'I was overcome by the hurt and sadness of my son being ignored by the very people he was related to,' says Sally. 'Their silence after Massimo had his spinal surgery was the final insult.'

It brought into sharp clarity who and what really mattered to them. Those who loved Massimo uncon-ditionally, who sat by his bed, always there to comfort Sally and Stephen and offer support, were the people they wanted in their lives. It was a small but dedicated group, which included Sally's parents, her brother, John, Massimo's carer, Siobhan, and his best friend, Jo. While Jo originally came into his life as a paid carer, during her free time she would come and visit him, lying by his side as they watched the same Wiggles episode over and over on his iPad.

'When you have a child who becomes terribly vulnerable due to illness, it is very comforting to see him surrounded by so much love,' says Sally. 'And it hurts so much more when he is rejected, because at the end of the day he is innocent – it's not as though he brought this awful disease on himself.'

Stephen was so incensed by the lack of acknowledge-ment of Massimo's plight from some of Sally's relatives, that in early April 2011 he wrote them a formal letter ending the relationship.

'Not everyone will agree with a difficult decision,' he says several years down the track. 'That is precisely what makes it difficult. I had lost all faith in them and during this time of crisis I didn't want to allow negativity into our home. We wanted to focus on diagnosing Massimo and this was just an unwelcome distraction.'

As if all this emotional stress wasn't enough, soon after Massimo returned home from spinal cord surgery, Stephen's father, Alfio, was rushed to hospital again, struggling to breathe with ongoing respiratory issues. If ever there was even the slightest doubt for having taken such a final action it was soon cast aside.

'I was sitting beside my gravely ill father in Emergency, as he rested after being stabilised with inhalers and nebulisers. My son was at home recovering from his surgery. We needed to save him and the bottom line was that you were either supporting him or you weren't. Massimo needed to be surrounded by friends and family who loved him unconditionally, in sickness and in health.'

Once stabilised, the nursing staff wheeled Alfio up to the ward. As they went to move him from the gurney to a bed, Stephen realised his father had slipped into a coma. A Code Blue alarm was raised and medical staff came running in. Stephen was asked to wait outside while the team worked on Alfio, who had gone into respiratory arrest.

'They rushed over a defibrillator trolley and the paddles came out. Then the doors to the room closed. I didn't need to see what happened next; I could hear it.'

After a few minutes, a senior respiratory consultant came out to talk to Stephen.

'He's in a serious state at the moment and we're going to try to stabilise him before hopefully moving him down to the Intensive Care Unit.'

Alfio was one of six siblings, most of whom still lived in Italy. That evening, Stephen called his cousin Antonella in Spoltore to tell her he didn't think Alfio was going to live past the weekend. He asked her to pass the news on to the rest of the family. On the Sunday, at around 5.30 pm, Stephen and Sally were in the kitchen getting dinner ready for the kids when the phone rang. Sally handed the phone to Stephen thinking it was probably the hospital calling. He went into their bedroom to take the call, expecting to hear either that his father had died, or a difficult decision needed to be made regarding whether or not to turn off the ventilator that was keeping him alive.

'Hello, Stephen?' It was a woman's voice on the other end.

'Speaking.'

'My name is Anna Maria.'

'Yes. How can I help you?'

'Well, this is going to sound strange, but I am your half-sister. They just called me from Italy to tell me that our father is in hospital.'

Stephen acknowledges now that a normal person would be thinking 'What the hell?!'

'At this point in time, though, with all that had been

going on with Massimo, the IVF, my mother's rapidly advancing Alzheimer's disease and the rift in Sally's family, I think if there had been a knock at the door and Darth Vader had been standing there saying, "I am your father", I probably would have invited him in for a drink and asked him how his plans for the new Death Star were coming along.'

When Stephen walked into the boys' room half an hour later, Sally was busy changing nappies. She was expecting the worst.

'Was that the doctor?'

Stephen kept a poker face. 'Don't worry. Dad's okay for now. Let's get the kids to bed and I'll explain once they're asleep.'

As soon as the twins were tucked into their cots, Sally turned her attention to Massimo. Stephen went to pour himself a glass of wine.

Massimo went to sleep quickly and Sally went out to the backyard, where she found Stephen nervously smoking a cigarette from a packet he was given by a friend at the hospital earlier. It was his second for the day, after many years of abstinence.

Sally stood on the back step staring at him.

'What's wrong?' she asked.

'Have a seat.'

'No. It's too cold,' Sally protested.

'Trust me. You need to sit down.'

Sally lowered herself onto the concrete step, hugging her knees with her arms, in a brace position for disaster.

'You know that call before? It wasn't the doctor. It was my half-sister, Anna Maria.'

The following day Stephen went to the hospital, where he had arranged to meet Anna Maria for the first time. He entered the building and waited patiently for the lift. The doors opened and he came face-to-face with actor Rachel Griffiths and her son.

'My jaw dropped. I thought you've got to be joking; not because she was a famous actress, but because she starred in the TV series *Brothers and Sisters*.'

In the opening episode of the show, Griffiths plays one of the daughters of a wealthy patriarch who has a heart attack and dies in his luxurious pool. Soon after, a secret second family emerges out of the woodwork. Life imitates art.

Stephen took the elevator up to the Intensive Care Unit and spoke to his dying father, who had started to regain consciousness.

'Someone called last night,' Stephen said.

His father stared at him with puffy eyes, looking confused.

'You've got some explaining to do. Who the hell is Anna Maria?'

'Oh, yes,' his father said quietly. 'Your sister. Do you like her?'

'Why didn't you tell me?'

'I don't know. It was no big deal.' Alfio paused. His chest was heaving and the heart monitor beeped rapidly.

'I wanted to tell you, but with everything going on with Massimo, the timing wasn't right.'

'Did you think when I told you it was vitally important for me to know about our whole family history, it might have been relevant?'

Stephen tried to get more information from his father, but couldn't push him because of the state of his health. Now wasn't the right time. After lunch, he went outside to meet Anna Maria alone. He felt completely disconnected from what should have been a touching moment – meeting his sister for the first time.

'I was severely depressed. I really didn't react to anything any more. If you had told me I had stage-four cancer and was going to die within six months I probably wouldn't have been too distraught. I simply couldn't take much more of living in the limbo of an unknown future for my little boy. I was completely exhausted, both mentally and physically and not thinking rationally. I didn't appreciate the significance of the new family at the time because I was so focused on diagnosing Massimo. Everything else felt like noise. It was a distraction to tell the story of our lives over and over. I also didn't know where I would find the strength to explain my father's secret life to all our friends and Sally's immediate family. I had been made a fool of and now it seemed a lot of time was going to be wasted setting straight my father's mess.

'I recognised Anna Maria immediately because she was the spitting image of my father. We didn't hug or do any of the things you might expect on such a momentous occasion. Instead we went straight into a small meeting room where I clinically explained what had happened to our father, how they were managing his condition and the likely grim prognosis. Then we went into our father's room together.'

Alfio opened his eyes to see his two adult children standing together at the foot of his bed.

'Okay,' he said matter-of-factly. 'So now you two have met. That's good.'

The next day, Stephen and Anna Maria returned to the hospital and had a longer conversation. Although they had nearly forty years of lost time to make up for, Stephen felt drained. The more he learned about his father's double life the more he felt disappointed for having given him a second chance. He was about to excuse himself and go home to bed when there was an awkward pause in the conversation.

'Hang on. There's more,' Anna Maria said. 'He came to Melbourne with his brother.'

'Oh, really? I didn't know that,' said Stephen. 'Which one? Edmondo, Tonino or Giulio?'

'No,' she said quietly, folding her napkin and looking down at the table. 'Evo.'

'What do you mean?' Stephen was floored. 'I've been to Italy. I've met the entire family. Who is Evo?'

'He had four brothers. You have another uncle you never knew about. He lived right here in Melbourne. You also have four first cousins you've never met.'

Stephen was furious. When Massimo became ill he had specifically asked his father if he knew of any family members who had neurological conditions, even making him call Italy to check.

'At no point did he tell us he had a brother in Australia who had so many children and grandchildren. When it was critical for Sally and me to know our entire family history, my father had sat on this information. He really crossed the line with that. I felt completely betrayed given the number of times I had been to Italy and no one had said anything. It turns out they had all been sworn to secrecy.'

It became apparent to Stephen that, whatever the reason for his secrecy, the only way his father had been able to keep the whole house of cards from falling down was to keep the families separate, but it came at such a heavy price. Even now, long after his father's death, Stephen has trouble forgiving him.

'If you place yourself in the mind of someone born in conservative 1920s Italy, it might make sense. I understand his thinking but don't agree with it and I don't imagine anyone would have cared less. I guess after so long it became easier to continue living a lie rather than telling the truth.'

Alfio had an electrical engineering background and retrained himself as an electrician in Australia, eventually working as a technician in the microbiology department at the University of Melbourne. While he was there he met Hilda, Stephen's mother, at a favourite university restaurant, Genevieve. She was a fiercely intelligent and beautiful woman who had studied computer science at the Royal Melbourne Institute of Technology and then completed a Master of Arts. She spoke seven languages fluently.

Stephen says, 'I think in his mind he'd moved on from a small town to a big city. He came from a traditional Italian Catholic family and wanted to keep up appearances, so he never divorced his first wife, Elizabeth. I ended up being his illegitimate son. Anna Maria almost had a nervous breakdown in 2009, trying to hold on to this secret. My sister and I were the collateral damage of our father's house of cards.'

The sad thing was that Stephen grew up alone – always wishing he'd had a large extended family. Ninety per cent of the time Christmas was spent with his mother and her old French au pair who had moved to Australia, not a child his age in sight.

Over the next fortnight, as Alfio recovered from his attack, Stephen spent an extraordinary amount of time speaking with Anna Maria, trying to piece together his father's parallel life. He was gobsmacked by the extent of his charade, which included forging a marriage certificate. Stephen discovered it tucked away in a filing cabinet where it had been kept for years. 'Unless you're looking for something, sometimes you just don't know it's there.'

Sally always jokes that Stephen missed his calling as an intelligence agent.

'Thank goodness we don't have any daughters,' she says.

'Their future boyfriends would never endure his interrogations. He's just like the retired CIA agent character Jack Byrnes, played by Robert De Niro in *Meet the Parents*. Stephen remembers minute details – people's faces, the watches they wear, the colour of their belt, but interestingly never names. If you asked him to describe a room he had stood in for a few minutes ten years ago he could list the number of light switches, power points, chairs, tables, doors – it's quite remarkable. His visual–spatial and auditory mind works at a different level; he sees patterns most people don't. Once he went to a twenty-first birthday party and randomly met someone who was introduced by first name only. Just from the guy's mannerisms and the way he laughed, he picked it was another friend's brother, whom he'd never met before.'

The strange thing was that Stephen had been living with his parents' secret right under his nose his entire life and never suspected anything. It never entered his head to ask why there were no wedding photos displayed around the house. He just assumed it was because they had parted ways. Anna Maria had kept Alfio's secret safe her entire life and only told her own family in 2009, when her children – considerably older than their newly found uncle Stephen – were already in their forties.

Now that Stephen knew his father's secret, things started falling into place. Back in 2004, Stephen had become involved with helping his mother with a property reparation claim, related to her family's wartime experience of living as a foreigner in Romania.

While on a business trip to Europe in 2008, he had travelled there to gather legal documents previously submitted to the Romanian courts. In Bucharest, he found two distant cousins of his mother who handed him a portfolio containing his parents' marriage certificate among the documents. He didn't notice then that the orientation of the record was incorrect – landscape instead of portrait. After Anna Maria's call Stephen went to the portfolio in his office and pulled out his parents' marriage certificate, dated 25/9/1967. It was so obvious to him in retrospect that it was a fake.

Sally was in a state of shock.

'It felt as though it was one thing happening after another. Yes, the dismissal of the family to protect Massimo was planned in advance and was a decision that we had taken together, but their reactions afterwards still hurt, especially when they mocked my family. Following all this, to be hit with Alfio's secret family out of the blue was a whole other thing. Life was starting to take on a cinematic feel. People often don't believe us when we tell them the stories.'

Anna Maria lives in North Melbourne, 300 metres from the Royal Children's Hospital where Massimo has been treated since 2008.

'We must have driven past, or parked almost in front of her house countless times,' muses Stephen. 'What was so striking was that she knew everything about me, including Massimo and the twins. She had photos, as well as magazine and newspaper articles about me that my father had given her.'

Anna Maria had always known about Stephen. Alfio left her mother back in the 1960s before meeting Stephen's mother, Hilda. They moved across town to the opulent suburb of Toorak, where they shared a two-bedroom apartment with Hilda's mother. After a while Stephen came along, but by the time he was six months old, Alfio had moved on again.

Alfio Damiani was a charming character, with a booming voice and handsome looks. He immigrated to Australia in 1954. It turns out that when he left Italy he was already married and had a five-year-old daughter – Anna Maria – both of whom he brought along with him. He set up a restaurant called Alfio's Bistro in the late 1970s, one of the first trendy Italian restaurants on Toorak Road, in the upmarket suburb of South Yarra.

'Alfio's was always overflowing back in the eighties,' says Stephen. 'If you ever had a coffee or hot chocolate from there, with a Baci on the side, chances are my father made it. I remember we had to call in advance, to make sure he'd be there before we turned up for dinner. Little did I know then, the reality was he was secretly juggling two families.'

It wasn't until Stephen was at university in 1993, that his father moved in with them after developing lung cancer. The doctors told them his condition was inoperable and gave him six to nine months to live. Hilda looked after him, going to great lengths to find alternative therapies, including intravenous vitamin infusions, papaya and shark cartilage extracts. Even though Stephen didn't necessarily agree with these treatments, the degree of effort his mother went to, and her determination and refusal to give up certainly rubbed off on him.

'My father had been absent for most of my life. I had no paternal guidance whatsoever as I was growing up. When I was obsessed with restoring my first car instead of paying attention to my studies, he went out of his way to encourage me. Rather than suddenly wanting to be a good father, he was trying to gain acceptance and make up for not being around for the past twenty years.'

A couple of weeks later, when Alfio was discharged from the rehabilitation hospital, Stephen didn't hold back in trying to extract some more information from him.

'The drive home should have taken ten minutes, but instead we went around in circles yelling at each other for two hours.'

'Just put a stone on it. That's it,' Alfio said.

'His father certainly didn't share any of Stephen's genes for overanalysing conversations,' says Sally. 'I worried that this chain of events was taking its toll on Stephen as he was essentially in the front line, copping it from every angle. He made the call to stand up to my family, to protect Massimo from being hurt. On top of that, not only was he dealing with a father who was now dying, he was also learning about a whole new family. I thought his mind was going to explode with all that was going on. Once Alfio was out of hospital and in a stable condition, I suggested he get away for a few days to clear his head, so he booked a short trip to Fiji just to disconnect from the craziness that our lives had become.'

Stephen's grandparents on his mother's side, Stepan and Arussiag Gurdikyan, were of Armenian descent and came from privileged backgrounds. They had servants and a nanny for their two daughters, and lived in a grand home in Istanbul. They emigrated to the city of Bucharest in Romania in 1937, after receiving numerous anonymous death threats. Stephen's mother, Hilda, was two years old and her sister, Laura, was six at the time. They never found out who sent those letters, but with war looming in the West, and with the genocide of Armenians by the Ottoman government only twenty years earlier, Stepan was concerned that one day something terrible might happen to his family. They lived through the war in Bucharest and set up a thriving textile business, which narrowly escaped being bombed.

After World War II, when the Iron Curtain fell, there was growing anti-foreigner sentiment in Romania. Secret police would intimidate the family and stalk their house day and night. They lived in fear of being arrested by the Romanian Securitate, under the guise of accusations that they exploited workers. The government used this as an excuse to expel Hilda and Laura from school. The family decided to leave Romania at the end of 1953, using their Turkish passports, because they were tipped off that the government was going to arrest Stepan. Without telling a soul, early one morning the whole family pretended to go for a walk, leaving all their belongings at home so as not to arouse suspicion. They stayed with a trusted Romanian family for a week and then caught a train from Bucharest to the seaside town of Constanta, where they bribed some port workers to arrange a meeting with the captain of a coal ship. They paid the captain handsomely to smuggle them out, hidden in a secret compartment.

After sailing for two days across the Black Sea, the Gurdikyans arrived in Istanbul. There they looked up a cousin who arranged a job for Stepan as the Director of the Armenian Hospital.

In 1954, Hilda moved to Paris to study law at the Sorbonne, and soon after to London to learn English. She wasn't enamoured with London, so when she heard about opportunities in Australia she decided to set sail for Melbourne in 1963. Once there, she saved enough money to pay for her parents' passage too. Sadly, her father, Stepan, died of lung cancer soon after their arrival, well before his grandson Stephen was born.

'Mum was a quiet achiever and adventurer,' says Stephen. 'She decided to leave and go it alone as a young woman on several occasions, but this was survival not pleasure. Despite being a nagging and overprotective mother, she was comfortable with letting me travel around North America on my own when I turned eighteen. She always wanted me to experience the things she didn't get the opportunity to. She was obsessed with me studying medicine, but I didn't have the slightest inclination or the marks. When I finished school, I was accepted into a

Bachelor of Aviation Engineering to train as a pilot, but she begged me not to take up the offer because she thought it was too dangerous. It's something I still regret not doing, although my astigmatism may have been a career-limiting factor anyhow.'

Hilda's mother lived with them from when Stephen was born. He was very close to his grandmother; she picked him up from school every day, prepared dinner and cared for him until his mother came home from work. She usually spoke Armenian or French to him, but made a huge effort to learn English by watching television and listening to news broadcasts. She loved Malcolm Fraser and Bob Hawke, and avidly followed their political debates. When Stephen was in Year 3 he remembers his grandmother dressing up, putting on her finest jewellery, applying makeup and standing in front of the television to talk to the Prime Minister and Leader of the Opposition. That was the first sign of the onset of Alzheimer's, which was to ravage her brain until her death in 1986, while Stephen was away at Year 8 camp.

Sally and Stephen first met at a wedding back in 1998. They headed out to a bar afterwards with a group of people, talking and dancing until late into the night. At the end of the evening Stephen gave her his number, hoping she would call, but when she finally plucked up the courage the timing was terrible.

'I was a fresh graduate working at IBM. We were all putting in ridiculous twenty-hour shifts in the final days before major bid submissions, but it was always fun. We were a young team of graduates who enjoyed working together, thriving in the chaos; we just got things done. It was around noon when Sally rang, and we were all frantically replacing pages in a bid still being reviewed and due across town at 2 pm. We had a ten-second conversation, which ran something like: "Hi. It's really nice to hear from you, but I'll have to call you back." We were all so stressed in the office; I remember the sales manager rolling a cigarette just before we all raced downstairs to load everything into an awaiting car, ready to whisk him off to submit the bid. He hopped into the front passenger seat with the cigarette hanging from his mouth, as we piled in the documents through the back door. After a short while we realised it was the wrong car, an identical Jeep Cherokee to the one waiting for him in front, with the driver sitting there speechless. In the end we made it with less than five minutes to spare.'

Stephen, completely exhausted, called Sally back as soon as he got home from work that afternoon and they arranged to go out on the following Saturday.

'We went out for a coffee and she told me her surname was Bakian. Her eyes nearly popped out of her head when I asked a question in Armenian. It was the first time I'd spoken the language since my grandmother had died twelve years earlier, but later it came in handy because I met with instant approval when I was introduced to Sally's Armenian grandmother.'

Stephen highly respected Sally's drive and motivation; she had studied business and marketing at Monash

University and started a graduate diploma of computing soon after he first met her.

'She had a good head on her shoulders. We could have robust conversations and really challenge one another. I saw that we shared similar attitudes when it came to working hard. There wasn't any sense of entitlement in Sally.'

They dated for two years and then on New Year's Eve 2000, Stephen popped the question on the spur of the moment, something so out of character for a man who likes to plan everything down to the tiniest detail.

'It just seemed like the right timing,' he says, smiling broadly. 'I didn't even have a ring. The following morning we went to tell Sally's parents and they asked if I'd like a coffee. I told them, "I need a Scotch!"'

Stephen and Sally were married two years later, in December 2002, soon after Stephen completed his MBA. Sally laughs when talking about it. 'You can bet that our wedding was meticulously planned – Stephen had a spread-sheet to manage it all, down to the last minute.'

Stephen's mother, Hilda, had longed for the day she would hold a grandchild in her arms, so soon after Massimo was born Stephen knew something was wrong with her.

'This should have been the most exciting day for her; she'd wanted a grandchild for years. But she just didn't seem excited when she came to visit Massimo at the hospital for the first time.'

Soon after, Stephen started to notice some very odd transactions in numerous family bank accounts. Tens of thousands of dollars were being taken out, with thirty balance requests over two days in the same location. Hilda's internet banking had been locked due to forgotten passwords and he was able to trace the withdrawals to ATMs at various gaming venues. He soon realised that she was also thousands of dollars behind in bill payments. He turned up at his parents' house to confront his father.

'It wasn't me,' Alfio replied. He sat poker-faced on the couch in the lounge room, watching CNN. Nine months of unpaid bills were spread out on the floor as Stephen tried to make sense of what was going on. Utilities and phone companies had been changed twice and there were multiple disconnection notices and letters from debt collectors. Stephen's mother was crying, wondering why this was all happening, saying she was stupid and hitting her head. She knew her mind was going.

'You've taken Mum by the hand and made her pull out thousands from bank accounts over the past six weeks!' he yelled at his father. 'You're clearly taking advantage of her memory going.'

'Oh, no,' his father said. 'We had expenses.'

'Stop the bullshit! Thousands have gone walkabout. You've gambled it away, haven't you? How could you be so irresponsible?'

Alfio shouted at his son, 'I can do what I want.'

'No you can't. Enough is enough. You wrecked her life, you were never around in my life until you were sick, and I am not going to let you hurt my son,' Stephen said, drawing the line.

From that point on, Stephen locked down the family's finances to protect his mother.

'I could have dealt with my father's forty-year clandestine life, but his shenanigans on top of everything were just too much to bear at times. Over the following three years, until his passing, we had a very cool relationship, even though I was always the "fixer" taking care of everything for him. He didn't appreciate how much time and effort it took to make the world work around him. He never realised what a financial, personal and professional toll he took on all of us. He outsourced all of that until the day he died.'

The last time Stephen saw his father was in early October 2011.

'By this stage we couldn't really be in a room together for more than a few minutes before we started arguing. He still insisted he had done no wrong, saying, "Maybe we spent fifty dollars on the pokies now and then" and claimed I was exaggerating despite having shown him the bank records. He couldn't see why I was so disappointed and hurt that he had lied to everyone for forty years, refusing to give any explanation; simply brushing me off and repeatedly telling me to "put a stone on it and move on".'

Stephen maintains that the only reason his father never brought the two families together was for self-preservation.

'He wasn't protecting anyone but himself. Maybe if I'd heard the word "sorry" in an unconditional context I might have let go, but there wasn't the slightest sense of remorse. He started shouting and swearing in front of Massimo. Sally and I both told him to lower his voice and have some respect, but he just waved his arm and dismissed us.

' "Oh! He doesn't understand anything," he yelled, brushing his grandson off as "retarded", without explicitly stating it.

' "You really don't care about anyone or anything but yourself any more, do you?" I said, standing in front of my father.'

Alfio stood up and stormed off, swearing in Italian.

'I didn't speak to him again, but I called Anna Maria and told her our father had gone mad and walked out. I asked her to keep an eye on him because he was having trouble breathing and to keep me posted. A week or so later, my mother's sister, Laura, who had moved to Australia in 2002, called and said he was struggling to breathe. I told her to call an ambulance right away and raced over to find him lying on the floor. There was no pulse and I started CPR, pumping his chest.'

The ambulance crew arrived within a minute, asking Stephen if he wanted them to try to resuscitate his father. He said yes and they immediately started inserting lines, clearing Alfio's throat and sticking electrodes onto his chest.

'I remember looking at my watch and thinking it's been fifteen minutes now. He's gone.'

Alfio's heart started again and he was taken to the hospital where Stephen's sister met them. Doctors explained that his kidneys weren't functioning, that too much damage had been done and he would never recover. Together, they made the call to stop all attempts to revive him. Stephen stood beside his father as he passed away within minutes of turning off the life support.

'In the end, it was his dual life that killed him – it sapped an enormous amount of energy from him. Anna Maria said he always complained of feeling like a "fugitive", running from his past. I don't think he ever wanted children, nor did he understand what it really meant to be a father; he thought the title was inherited through genes, not something that was earned. After everything we've been through over the past few years, he epitomised how outdated this notion of family is in the 21st century.'

Chapter 10

MISSION ACCOMPLISHED

Somewhere in their son's data was the answer Stephen and Sally were looking for, but finding it was proving elusive. Massimo had an unknown variation or mutation in a gene not previously associated with a Leukodystrophy, and they needed to search wider rather than focus on known conditions; that had been the real purpose for sequencing his genome in the first place. Stephen approached Callum Bell, program leader at the National Center for Genome Resources (NCGR) – a non-profit research institute and one of Illumina's partners based in Santa Fe – and arranged to have the data analysed further. Bell consulted with his colleague Stephen Kingsmore, the Chief Science Officer, who suggested analysing Massimo's entire genome first and only going ahead with the trio analysis if indicated.

'Again, no one could guide us on potential results because it hadn't been performed locally, and perhaps only a handful of times internationally with limited success,' says Stephen. 'In theory, single-genome analysis would identify all of the known and unknown variations compared to a baseline genome that might be causing Massimo's condition. In reality what would come out was anyone's guess. We hoped it wasn't going to be a staggering number.'

Stephen was always planning the next steps, even if they weren't needed, so they would never grind to a halt and need to rebuild momentum.

'The minute we hit a dead end we needed a contingency option ready. We couldn't afford any down time. There was either going to be a smoking gun or we would have to take the next step, which was to run trio analysis that required both parental genomes to be sequenced. This meant another $20,000 to $30,000 in sequencing, plus at least the same again for the analysis – it was getting expensive but that was where the science was taking us.'

Sally and Stephen requested a meeting with the local medical and genetics team from the Royal Children's Hospital and Victorian Clinical Genetics Services – George McGillivray, David Amor, Rick Leventer and Kate Pope – to seek their guidance. According to all of Stephen's research the next step, if required, had never been performed on one undiagnosed paediatric patient and would be costly, so he really wanted their technical direction before committing. Rounding up so many people to be in the same place, at the same time, was tricky.

'Finally we had everyone in the room together for our "Come-to-Jesus Meeting",' says Stephen. 'Our intention was to update everyone on the progress with NCGR, discuss the possible outcomes and seek an independent opinion on the best way forward. I was looking for validation of our strategy and approach. After we all exchanged greetings and sat down the opening words came as a surprise: "We thought we'd let you chair the meeting." '

This was quite an honour for Stephen, but at the time he felt like someone had just handed over the controls to a plane for his first solo flight.

'I was a little startled by this opening,' says Sally. 'But Stephen quickly found his feet. The funny thing was he would keep apologising for his lack of knowledge, which was just crazy, given how much he had upskilled himself over the previous eighteen months.'

It was agreed the phased strategy of single genome and then familial trio genome analysis was theoretically sound, but it was blue-sky research and no one was sure what would come out at the end. What was clear, though, was if the single-genome analysis from NCGR yielded thousands, hundreds or even dozens of leads there were no local resources to analyse it further.

Four weeks later, the number of possible variations in Massimo's DNA came back as a staggering 11,481 across a total of 5726 genes. One or more of these variations was almost certainly the cause of Massimo's condition, but the figure was far too large to be anything meaningful to work with. Callum Bell had coined the term 'genome vertigo' for this overwhelming amount of data.

Stephen had known from the outset both Sally's and his own genomes would eventually need to be sequenced, hoping that comparing them to Massimo's DNA blueprint through a series of complex algorithms would remove the common variations. If Sally or Stephen were carrying these variations yet weren't affected by the disease, then it pretty much ruled them out. They had to find something unique in Massimo: mutations that may have been transferred as a combination from both of them. The way to do this was through a process called *familial trio genome analysis*, something that had been in Stephen's mind since Paris. It was going to involve a differential analysis on the trillions of different possible combinations.

'This was our July 1969 moon shot. It was our last chance to achieve a diagnosis,' says Stephen.

Aside from the enormous financial and technical challenges they faced, the greatest limitation was that they only had one affected patient: Massimo. If there had been a cohort of a dozen or more children with similar symptoms and MR imaging changes as Massimo, it would have made it far easier to pinpoint a common variation causing the disease.

While NCGR could align and identify genetic variants or deviations from the baseline human genome in Massimo's DNA, they no longer provided the service of 'genome annotation'. That is, they could identify changes in Massimo's genes, but were unable to help determine what those genes actually do. This was due to lack of demand at the time, as well as the prohibitive licence cost of accessing reference libraries with lists of variant-to-disease associations. Local genetic health services had neither the experience nor the resources. The real challenge now was to find someone who was willing and able to perform this trio analysis.

Faced with brick walls on every side, Stephen simply tightened his belt and set forth on yet another research project of his own. Long before embarking on the journey of mapping Massimo's genome, Stephen had begun immersing himself in a self-education program in genomics. The first thing he did was order an eBook of *Genetics For Dummies* online. Soon after that he bought another, which he also read cover to cover – *Bioinformatics For Dummies*.

'I know these weren't exactly Reed Elsevier scientific titles,' he acknowledges. 'But I didn't have three years to educate myself. I needed to bring my knowledge up to a sufficient level quickly, in order to understand the latest research papers. Then I would be able to ask the right questions of the right people. I just needed to speak the same language as the experts, to allow me to make the best decisions for my son.'

Stephen went to see Leah at the clinic by himself one day.

'He walked into my room clutching a wad of papers to his chest, wide-eyed and sporting a half-smile I had gradually come to recognise as a shield for his underlying anxiety,' she says. 'He sat down beside my desk and spread the bunch of journal articles out in front of me. I must have looked like a stunned chipmunk because his nervous grin turned into a broad smile.'

Stephen began telling her how he needed a bioinformatics guru to align, analyse and interpret a familial trio of genomes. It would require all the data they had already generated from mapping Massimo's genetic blueprint and now they needed to sequence their own genomes for the exercise. He had all sorts of options in mind, including doing the job himself.

Stephen says, 'On the National Human Genome Research Institute website I found links to presentations and lists of attendees from the recent American Society of Human Genetics (ASHG) conference in Washington DC and reached out across the globe. I even watched several videos from the conference that had been posted on YouTube, to hear the questions being asked and to see who was asking them. Some experts replied to my emails politely, saying that what I was suggesting wasn't going to be possible right now with only one affected patient. Others took the time to make some valuable suggestions, pointing me in the right direction to someone who might be able to help. Some didn't respond at all.'

Stephen even thought about developing a smartphone app.

'It would download small chunks of our genetic data which would be analysed in the background. It would follow a similar principle to the SETI@home project.'

The SETI (Search for Extraterrestrial Intelligence) project, established in 1999, was founded by Frank Drake and Carl Sagan to analyse radio signals from outer space via people's personal computers.

'You would download a screen saver from the SETI@home project website and packets of data from radio telescopes around the world to analyse,' explains Stephen. 'Every time your screen saver activated it would sift through the data searching for anomalies and show visuals of the radio frequencies being analysed. A detection would provide evidence of extraterrestrial technology. Maybe I worked with geeks, but I remember half our floor had it running on their screens at lunch and we'd jokingly ask in the lifts if anyone had found E.T. that day.'

To date it has attracted over five million volunteer participants worldwide.

'Just imagine how many phones this could be run on in parallel these days; the ultimate distributed computing platform.'

Leah sat with her arms crossed, looking alternately at the floor and her watch. She didn't have the slightest clue what Stephen was talking about and found herself wondering if he was finally losing the plot. Stephen persisted, despite her obvious body language.

'The answer is there in the data. We just need a way to analyse it. This is so out there, it will surely raise awareness and interest in our mission to diagnose Massimo. Someone will come out of the woodwork to help.'

Stephen even wanted to set up an XPRIZE, notifying

researchers around the world about his mission. He wanted to approach Illumina, with the aim of asking them to donate a few whole-genome sequences to the winning team. As he spoke, Leah furtively typed *XPRIZE* into Google, hoping he wouldn't notice. 'XPRIZE is the global leader in the creation of incentivized prize competitions. Our mission is to bring about radical breakthroughs for the benefits of humanity, thereby inspiring the formation of new industries . . .'

Leah recalls: 'I'd just frozen a wart off the previous patient's nose, and an impatient elderly lady had shuffled into the waiting room for her regular prescriptions and blood pressure check. I had only just barely got my head around what a genome was – wading through the journal articles Stephen had plied me with over the previous eighteen months, trying to keep up with his exponential rise in knowledge and expertise in the field. I'm sure at times he must have felt like I was borrowing his watch to tell him the time. But when he started waxing lyrical about *bioinformatics*, I have to fess up – he had truly left me for dead.'

One evening, Leah arranged to meet up with Erica Sontheimer, a writing colleague who worked for a cutting-edge literary journal called *Griffith REVIEW*. Erica had recently edited a piece Leah had written about how physicians have a tendency to develop 'tunnel vision of the soul' – an inability to read the nuances in a patient's narrative – something Leah felt she was often guilty of herself.

Leah was telling Erica about the Damiani family as a case in point; and of some colleagues she had spoken to who were tending to dismiss their ideas for further investigation of their son as pure science fiction.

'We met in the cosmopolitan Melbourne suburb of East St Kilda, where by day you usually need to elbow your way past sturdy little Russian ladies, beefy Australian labourers wearing shorts and boots, and Hasidic Jews rushing in and out of bagel bakeries and continental delicatessens. That evening, though, the street lay deserted; we walked up and down trying to find a café that was still open so we could sit and have a chat. We ended up at a table rammed against the front window of a falafel joint, sharing a pot of mint tea and a stale piece of baklava. It was the first time we'd met. I was the mother of three school-aged children and she was in her mid-thirties and recently married. She's an American and had followed her husband and his career across the Pacific Ocean to settle in Brisbane. We dived straight in, as girls will, sharing stories.'

Erica told Leah about growing up in Gettysburg, Pennsylvania, and of studying physics at university. She said she had always had a passion for writing and literature and in her twenties worked mostly in the not-for-profit arts sector, while also moonlighting as a yoga teacher. She was also a part-time marketing associate for Talking Eyes Media, a non-profit media company dedicated to advocating positive social change on pressing American issues such as the medically uninsured, aged care and more.

The conversation swiftly turned to stories of their previous lives and loves. 'We chatted about crazy adventures as single women, stories of our mutual lifetime love affair with New York City, a city I told her felt as if it was filled with a population of highly strung, neurotic, creative types who buzzed around from one exciting project to the next like bees, drunk from fields of beautiful flowers. We talked about movies and books, theatre and dodgy men in Amsterdam and Sydney. And we laughed to think how settled our inner "wild girls" had become, both now living in suburbia, happily married.

'I don't know what prompted me that evening to tell Erica the story of Sally and Stephen's journey, and then, as an afterthought, ask her if she knew anyone who worked in bioinformatics. I said it almost as a half-joke: "So, I don't suppose you happen to know any bioinformatics gurus, do you?"'

Erica stared at Leah with intelligent blue eyes, her eyebrows raised. Silver earrings dangled from her earlobes.

'Well, actually, my husband, Ryan, is a post doc fellow in bioinformatics.'

Leah looks back on that moment now as if it were frozen in time. 'It had been a nonchalant question. I was a fisherman sitting in a leaky wooden rowboat, casting a fifty cent line and lure into the middle of the ocean, hoping to catch a whale.'

'I wonder whether Ryan might be interested?' Erica mused.

*

When Ryan Taft was a five-year-old boy in Santa Barbara, he showed his parents a picture he had drawn of a water-powered car and told them he wanted to be an inventor.

'I was intrigued and inspired by people who make something out of nothing. It was so cool to conjure up things.'

Ryan used to take apart broken answering machines and blenders, trying to understand the process that went into making them.

'I knew there was power in that knowledge,' he says. 'One day my uncle did a mean thing – he brought three balls into our house and bet me I couldn't learn to juggle by morning. I stayed up all night and figured it out.'

Ryan started at the University of California, Davis, as a political science major on a full scholarship. 'I loved pure science, but I was determined to change the world. I'd even met the then Secretary of State, Madeleine Albright. I threw myself into philosophy and calculus classes.'

He lasted a year before telling his parents: 'This is horrible.'

He called a friend's mother who worked in a lab at UCD, to see if he could visit her. She offered him a job washing scientific instruments and by the end of that summer he was hanging out with chemists.

'One of the guys who held two PhDs wrote a synthesis equation up on a white board in the lab and they all started discussing it. I interrupted and, a little shyly, asked if he had missed a bond in one of the equations. They all stared at me, gobsmacked. It was then I realised: "I get this".'

Ryan fell straight into a research job at UCD, not far from Sacramento, and soon moved to a lab in San Francisco.

'My philosophy at the time was, "Why would I go to class to learn things people already know, when I could go into the lab and learn something entirely new?"'

Ryan had always wanted to work in paediatrics, but to avoid having to make a decision about applying for medical school he kept working in the lab.

'At the end of the day, I felt it was possible I could cut more roads into new territory and push more boundaries as a scientist rather than a clinician.'

As an undergraduate, Ryan spent his spare time working on his own idea that the importance of 'junk DNA', or the portions of a genome sequence that have no known biological function, was being overlooked by the scientific community. When the entire human genome was first mapped, less than 3 per cent was seen to contain coded information used to make crucial proteins. What was the other 97 per cent doing? The role of the rest of the DNA, referred to as 'junk DNA', was a total mystery. Ryan developed a hypothesis that the amount of junk DNA in a cell is correlated with how complex an animal is. This so-called junk DNA is a complex evolutionary system, which is actually vital for life and development.

'I was convinced I was onto something. I spent nights and weekends working on it.'

He was determined to un-junk 'junk DNA', knocking on many top scientists doors with his theories.

'I was literally getting laughed out of people's offices,' he says. 'But then I came across the work of John Mattick, who was saying the same thing, albeit from a different angle. I sent him a paper and pretty soon I got a National Science Foundation grant to go and work with him in Brisbane.'

Nowadays, the debate about junk DNA is shifting. The question is no longer one of 'Is junk DNA important?' – rather, the issue is how vital a role does it play?

'If genes themselves are the kind of eye-beams of a building, fundamental to the structure and function-ality,' explains Ryan, 'then junk DNA has proven to be its wiring, light switches, desks and internet cables. It is where all regulatory information lives. It deter-mines how genes are turned on and off and under which conditions.'

Colleagues he met at the University of Queensland's Institute for Molecular Bioscience, such as Marcel Dinger (now Head of Kinghorn Centre for Clinical Genomics at the Garvan Institute), were edgy and smart and they all bounced ideas off each other. John Mattick (now head of the Garvan Institute of Medical Research), a bit of a maverick genius who led the team, was just the mentor Ryan had been looking for. John had had an illustrious career as a scientist and gave Ryan the freedom to pursue his own creative ideas.

A couple of days after Leah's meeting with Erica, Sally popped into her clinic to pick up a script for Baclofen, a medication that helped stop the painful muscle spasms that woke Massimo up crying several times a night. Leah told Sally about her meeting with Erica and casually asked if she and Stephen would be interested in speaking to her husband Ryan, sensing for some reason that it would be really worthwhile that they connect. Sally went home and spoke to Stephen about it and that evening Leah sent an email introducing Stephen and Sally to Ryan Taft.

Within two hours Ryan had replied, elaborating on his background and explaining that his PhD had been awarded the Dean's Award for Outstanding Theses. The previous year he had been a finalist in two categories of the Australia Museum Eureka Prizes. He wrote:

My current work is focused on using the latest 'next generation' sequencing technologies to investigate everything from how genes are turned on and off, to discovering novel genetic mutations. I've been published in a number of leading journals, including Nature Genetics, Nature Structural & Molecular Biology, RNA, Cell Cycle, Neuro-Oncology *and others. We're currently in the process of setting up the University of Queensland Clinical Genomics Sequencing facility, and collaborate with scientists worldwide.*

I fear the paragraph above may make me look like an egomaniac – but I mention all of that only because Erica said you may have some genetic data pertaining to Massimo's condition that needs to be analysed. If I were in your shoes, and was considering handing that over to someone,

I would want to know that the data would be in very competent hands.

    Best regards,

    Ryan

'This was it,' says Ryan. 'This was the golden opportunity to apply what I had been studying. It was just what I had been waiting for.'

Stephen replied immediately and they organised to speak by phone the following evening.

'I remember being nervous,' says Ryan. 'I was stepping into a space where I was doing this by myself. I was just some guy and I wanted to make sure I could manage to keep Stephen's expectations at a realistic level. Turned out he was a very smart man who'd already done a ton of homework before he came to speak to me. He understood the problem and what he was hoping to do was bring together the right people to work in collaboration. He was sensible and tried to be objective. When a friend back in the US asked me about him later, I said, "You'll love him. He's one of us." By that I meant that he was willing to make things happen; he wasn't afraid to dream big. I love that disposition; that's what gets things done in this world. He wasn't crazy at all. For him it was a matter of risk mitigation – there was no increased risk to Massimo with all this, after all. And above all, what I liked was that Stephen wasn't prepared to give up. He was a bulldog. Well, he had to be of course – it was his kid we were talking about.'

Stephen and Ryan chatted for over an hour. Ryan only asked a few questions about Massimo.

'The data was the data. The presentation and nature of the patient's symptoms was irrelevant at the time. I really needed to separate the raw data from the clinical side of things; besides, I assumed his illness was genetic in origin. We were looking for something that stood out in his genome, or broke it apart.'

This approach also helped Ryan put a little distance between himself and the Damiani family, so he could remain clear-headed. Nonetheless, it was difficult to stay detached.

'I don't feel like I really had a choice. How could I say no to this guy whose son was dying? I couldn't get off the phone without saying yes.'

At the time, Ryan felt he was a kind of blank slate, in that he had nothing to lose by trying to help out. Stephen had tapped into that aspect of Ryan's personality that is fiercely determined to solve a problem. He harnessed the same kind of determination and focus he had shown as a little boy learning overnight how to keep three balls up in the air simultaneously.

'Once I'd said yes to Stephen, I couldn't let go of it. I knew what the data was, that it's not hard. It was an exciting problem. I knew this was the future and the potential that this data held to help these people. It fulfilled my wish of sitting somewhere on the borderlands of science and medicine. And now, as a father myself looking back on this, it was a no-brainer.'

'Ryan and Stephen were two magnets being joined together,' says Sally, recalling their first conversation. 'They shared the same drive. If there was no known way to do something they would figure it out.' She feels their tenacity and the strong connection between them helped drive the project.

Looking back on their first phone call, Stephen laughs. 'I could tell neither of us coped well with constraints that could easily be overcome with common sense. What we were proposing to do posed absolutely no danger to Massimo; we were just analysing data on a computer. I simply wanted to get on with it. We were looking at losing our son and without a diagnosis we could not help him. Every second counted.'

At first, keeping a professional distance, Ryan only asked Stephen a few questions about Massimo. Sequencing Sally's and Stephen's genomes to make a trio with Massimo's was going to take months. Working on the premise that DNA in affected cells is different from DNA in normal cells, Ryan thought the process could be sped up if they analysed the cells taken when Massimo had his spinal cord untethered.

At the same time, Professor Marjo van der Knaap in the Netherlands had raised the question around the diagnosis of 'mitochondrial disorders', a fault in the energy-producing apparatus of affected cells. Confirming this would mean liver and muscle biopsies, an arduous and painful procedure. Given their hopes to find a diagnosis through Ryan's analysis of their three genomes, Stephen and Sally were very reluctant to put Massimo under any more difficult procedures.

'Even if it did turn out that the cause of Massimo's illness was mitochondrial, the only intervention at the time would have been to give him Co-Enzyme Q10 supplements to help promote cell growth and maintenance. He was already taking them in small doses anyway. Besides, if we were to go ahead with the genome trio analysis, biopsies would be unnecessary; any mitochondrial disorder would pop up as a defective gene on the blueprint if this was the cause of Massimo's symptoms.'

In the months following the birth of the twins, Sally and Stephen started to see a real shift in Massimo's disposition. The scared, anxious boy he had become over the months following his diagnosis was fast disappearing and being replaced by a happy, curious and cheeky child. They continued to flood Massimo with therapy to help him develop as much as possible. Every gain, no matter how small, was celebrated.

'It was a sunny spring morning when we arrived at our music class held in a church hall,' says Sally. 'Massimo and I had been attending this class for over a year and his instructor, Tim, had a wonderful knack of making sure Massimo was always engaged in the class and connecting with the other children. When we first started, Massimo spent a lot of the time huddled in my lap, not even looking at Tim. Now that he had gained his newfound independence by being able to kneel up on his own, he was able to sit up like the other kids in the class and, with a little assistance from me, either helping him shake some maracas or holding him to dance around, he could participate in the whole class. We all sat around in a semi-circle on the floor for the class with Tim seated in the front, often playing his guitar. At the end of this particular class, while Tim was singing his farewell song Massimo crawled up to the front and climbed into Tim's lap to play the guitar with him. Most of the group had been with us when we started and there wasn't a dry eye among the mothers there, all of us so proud of Massimo for having the confidence to do what he did and endeared by the special bond that Massimo still has with Tim.

'Second to music, Massimo's other love was the iPad. We were amazed at how fast he took to it. After a few demonstrations from Stephen and me he quickly figured out how to recognise icons for the applications he wanted. He learned to scroll through the screens and interact on a basic level with the application. He would whoop with delight as he pressed the icon for the video player and a host of his favourite movies came up. He could choose one – usually his favourite Wiggles episode – and start it by himself.'

Sally and Stephen now faced some new challenges. When Massimo was first diagnosed and they thought they were going to lose him within a short space of time, they couldn't help but mollycoddle him.

'We attended to every whim, anticipating his needs before he even had an opportunity to express them,' says Sally. 'As Massimo began stabilising and the veil of fear that he would be slipping out of our lives at an early stage was lifting, we needed to start letting go. He needed the opportunity to develop appropriate ways of communicating that others could understand. In some ways, as awful as it felt, we let him know that he was not the centre of the universe.'

Addressing some of Massimo's inappropriate behaviours was as much a learning experience for Stephen and Sally as it was for him.

'I remember one afternoon in particular,' says Sally, 'I stood watching him lying on the lounge-room floor screaming because I wouldn't give him a chocolate before his dinner. Just as I was about to cave in, he stopped crying and ate his meal. I gave him the chocolate afterwards. All parents teach their children about manners and right and wrong behaviours. Massimo and I just had to do it a little differently. Letting his behaviour spiral out of control meant his participation in social settings would be limited even further than it already was.'

Most parents find it difficult to pull away from their young child and give them the opportunity to do things on their own. As the twins grew older, becoming increasingly mobile and vocal, it became more challenging for Stephen and Sally to divide their attention among the three children. To their surprise, Massimo started to do things for himself, reaching for a nearby bottle of water or happily playing with a toy on his own.

'The twins helped rebalance our household,' says Sally. 'It's hard to know what life would have been like without them. Would I have given Massimo the opportunity to try things on his own if it had just been the two of us and I had the time to compensate for any of his unmet needs? It had become such an ingrained and natural reaction. I still find myself reaching for a bottle of water and handing it to Massimo if he so much as flutters his eyelids, barely allowing him the opportunity to express what he is after. He usually readily accepts, reaffirming that my sixth sense about his need was correct. But I'm instantly racked with guilt for robbing him of the opportunity to communicate his needs to me. It is all well and good that we are both so attuned to him, but what would happen if we weren't around? Would he be able to communicate what he needs to others?'

The stability in Massimo's condition also meant that they had to start planning again. At the onset of his illness no one expected Massimo to live beyond his toddler years. Now this was becoming more and more likely, Sally and Stephen had to think about choosing the right school for him. Despite the slight improvement in skills, Massimo was still significantly disabled. He was unable to walk or talk, and needed help with feeding, dressing and toileting. Stephen and Sally were also uncertain of his intellectual abilities.

'The realisation that Massimo would be attending school sparked a whole new wave of fears and emotions,' says Sally. 'Would he be better off in a special or mainstream school? We tried to put ourselves in Massimo's shoes. If we were to send Massimo to a special school, having misjudged his intellectual abilities, would he get bored and frustrated? Conversely, if he went to a main-stream school, would he feel different and isolated from the rest of the class? How would we find the right aide to support him? Would he be able to keep up with the curric-ulum? We agonised over these scenarios for three years, well before he even attended kindergarten.'

Sally returned to work ten months after the twins were born. She started with a new firm in the corporate strategy team of a large Australian organisation. It took a while before the logistics of juggling a full-time job and three children ran smoothly. Everything had to be scheduled and planned and there was no room for leeway. She felt as if she were constantly walking a tightrope.

'About a year into my new job I was given the oppor-tunity to lead a major program of work, which meant taking on a significant amount of additional responsibility and a whole lot of staff. With this additional responsibil-ity came extra hours and new bosses with major demands. I soon realised that even though certain people espoused the importance of family and work–life balance, what they said and what they did was not consistent. My days at the office got longer and longer. When I'd get home, Stephen and I would make dinner and put the kids to bed, and then I'd turn the computer back on and work on into the night. Once again, my mum was a constant support to me through this period, along with Stephen who never complained about the long hours. I was determined to maintain my flexibility to come and go as I needed, to be there for Massimo's therapy and medical needs. I would start work late once a week after attending therapy with Massimo, and would meet Stephen or my mother at the Children's Hospital to attend medical appointments. The extra hours at night, or early in the morning, were my way of proving that I could be trusted to still get all of the work done, despite my absences. I didn't know how to be anything other than a conscientious worker.'

Sally's new perspective helped her with all the juggling.

'It meant that I no longer focused on trivia. Things that years ago may have been a disaster in my eyes, such as an error in a spreadsheet or a bad meeting with my boss, seemed insignificant compared to the challenges mounting at home. I found it a lot easier to move through things and oddly enough was more productive than ever before.'

She also knew that by working she was giving Stephen the time he needed to persevere with the diagnosis. The family motto had inadvertently become 'divide and conquer', but even though they were comfortable with this approach to their lives, it didn't stop others from having an opinion.

'Working mothers can be such a polarising topic, with those on both sides holding strong views. This is where I think the sisterhood lets itself down. I don't know why we spend so much time and energy passing judgement on mothers who do or do not work. As far as I am concerned, there is no magic formula or right answer. If a woman's particular situation means she needs to work, whether it is to pay the bills or just for her own sanity, the key issue is how to balance it with family life. For us it is about making every minute count. Whether it is at work, ensuring that I get as much done in my day so that I am not bringing work home to complete, or when I am at home with the kids giving them 100 per cent and not taking calls or checking emails. I have to admit that I am not a natural planner. With only myself and Stephen to worry about for so long, I was never one to write a list and managed to keep things in my head. This is now near impossible, so I have had to learn to love lists. It also helps when your husband is a born organiser. When I feel like there are too many variables to coordinate, he manages to churn out a logical plan off the top of his head. While it hasn't always been the case, I have learned to leverage this skill rather than try to replicate it.'

Ryan coined the new project PLD – Poor Little Dude. Within a month everything slowly began to fall into place. He wrote to the University of Queensland ethics department asking about any issues he needed to consider before setting out to analyse the genomes of Massimo and his parents. In a return email, they enquired if Ryan knew of anyone else who was able to do this project; would the family be able to get it done anywhere outside of a research facility? He told them he didn't think so and was surprised, yet delighted, when they wrote back telling him he might actually have an ethical obligation to do the work. Soon after he was awarded formal ethics approval.

'At that point we were off to the races!'

Ryan started the analysis using only Massimo's DNA, but ended up with too much 'noise' in the genome – lots of candidate genes popped up that might have been the cause of his symptoms, however he had no way of narrowing it all down. The publicly available data was sparse – he needed Massimo's parents' genomes to separate the signal from the noise. Since this was a genetic disease, and all Massimo's DNA had come from his parents, Ryan had to find what was different in Massimo's genome compared to Sally's and Stephen's. He turned to Illumina's representatives in Brisbane, and asked for help sequencing Sally and Stephen, assuring them that if the project were to be successful, it would be a terrific help for the Damiani family.

'I had no thoughts of anything beyond Massimo,' he says. 'I just wanted to get him a diagnosis. Once I took on the case I felt like I had signed a contract with Stephen. I would try at least as hard as he had to get Massimo's answers.'

Illumina suggested Ryan use one of their newest machines at the university. He spoke with the sequencing manager, and soon everyone was on-board and excited to help. Ryan also managed to persuade Illumina to supply $12,000 worth of reagents, the key substances consumed in the chemical reactions required to prepare DNA for sequencing.

'Illumina really wanted to see Massimo get a diagnosis,' he says. 'They were emotionally invested straight away. We'd had a long history of collaboration on many other research projects, so the local Illumina team was willing to take a chance on me, hoping that I might actually be able to pull this off. They also knew that if we were able to do this, it would be a big win for the technology.'

Ryan had the reagents shipped to his lab and was all set to start sequencing, when he realised delays within the university system would mean they would be slowed down. Stephen didn't want to lose momentum, and offered to further subsidise the effort to move things quickly, and with the help of Illumina they enlisted another company – Macrogen, based in Seoul – to perform all the sequencing at speed. Ryan sent them the reagents and they got all the data back to him within weeks.

Now he had a trio to work with, but no one could tell him what they were actually looking for.

'So, I decided to look at everything.'

This meant he looked at single base changes in genes, larger amplifications and deletions, copy number variants, as well as big structural changes.

'I spent lots of long nights and weekends at it. I think I was becoming borderline obsessed. I was convinced the answer was hidden in there somewhere – I just had to find it. I was searching for those few key differences between Massimo, Sally and Stephen.'

Erica remembers the many times Ryan would race out of the home office with delight, saying, 'I think I've got it!' She would give him a little hug and say, 'That's great, honey! Now have a snack.' He'd head straight back to his laptop for a few more hours and inevitably crawl back out into the kitchen late at night, disappointed. 'Nope, that wasn't it.'

'It was just a big differential analysis,' Ryan says. 'I slowly eliminated all likely candidates until I was left with just two genes – and only one of those was a perfect biological fit. It was a gene called DARS.' To Ryan, DARS made sense. The cousin of a similar gene already implicated in another Leukodystrophy (DARS2), DARS was expressed in the central nervous system, and when he did some complex computer modelling he found that the mutations sat in the most important part of the gene – a region called 'the active site'.

'I really thought I had it that time, so I wrote up the report. I was happy with the result, and confident that the work was solid, but I was nervous. I felt like I was putting my neck on the line at this point. The evidence, by all accounts, was still weak. But I was sure that this made more sense than anything else anyone had come up with. This was the best bet.'

Early in the evening on Saturday, 10 December 2011, a message from Ryan popped up on Stephen's smartphone: *Sent*. Stephen knew exactly what this meant – the trio analysis report had been forwarded. Ryan had to send it to a doctor first because it was a research report, not a clinical diagnosis. He needed a clinical intermediary. The minutes ticked away slowly as Stephen waited anxiously. He sent a message to Leah: *Please check your email – it's urgent.* Leah opened her computer and there it was in front of her. She immediately forwarded the report from Ryan. Seconds later, it arrived in Stephen's inbox.

'Embedded in the email was a link to download,' says Stephen. 'This was the trio analysis report we had been working so hard to achieve for almost two-and-a-half years. The children were all in bed and I sat at my desk for an hour reading every single word of this complex twenty-eight-page scientific paper.'

When he finished he raced down the hallway to tell Sally. 'It's solid. I think he's done it; I think he's got it.'

They had achieved a miracle. A plan conceived by a stubborn father and executed by a young, driven scientist on a shoestring budget, had potentially cracked the code of Massimo's DNA to identify the faulty gene. When Stephen excitedly forwarded the email to specialists around the world he was expecting high-fives and champagne corks to start popping immediately.

Instead the report was met with silence.

Chapter 11

WE NEED ANOTHER
MASSIMO

Ryan's analysis identified two variations, at different locations in Massimo's DARS gene. The DARS gene had never previously been associated with disease in humans. This was a new finding and everyone who received the report was confounded, needing time to digest the significance of the result. Sally and Stephen each carried one of these variations, which did not affect their own health. However, it was the unique combination inherited in Massimo, known as a compound heterozygous mutation, which was potentially causing his illness.

Two days before Christmas, out of frustration at the lack of response, Ryan shared the results with a trusted colleague and got him to run the data through an independent analysis pipeline. The results were the same, predicting the mutations in the DARS gene as the ones causing Massimo's disease.

Eventually the responses from specialists came through, which were highly praising of the report but raised an inconvenient truth:

$n = 1$

They only had one child in the sample. In order to prove that they had finally found the gene causing Massimo's illness, they had to show supporting results in one or more other studies. They needed more patients.

'It really knocked the wind out of our sails, but Ryan and I both knew that this was the next essential step,' says Stephen.

One option was to set up a research project to create a genetically engineered mouse in which the DARS gene would be inactivated, or 'knocked out'. Knockout mice are vital for studying the role of genes whose functions have not been determined. Disrupting the DARS gene in a mouse and observing any differences from normal behaviour or physiology might indicate its probable function.

Mice and humans share virtually the same set of genes. On average, the protein-coding regions of mouse and human genomes are 85 per cent identical – some genes are 99 per cent identical while others are only 60 per cent. In addition, mouse anatomy and physiol- ogy strikingly resembles a human's. The problem is, though, that mouse models are expensive ($250,000), time-consuming, and at the end of the day it's still only a mouse – there is always a gap in its applicability to human beings.

The preferred option was to find one or more affected children with a similar constellation of symptoms and MRI patterns as Massimo, and identify the same variations in the DARS gene. This would be a real game-changer.

Back in January 2011, while Stephen was scouring the internet on one of his 'Googling Missions', as Sally came to call them, he had stumbled across the Myelin Disorders Bioregistry Project. It was a research project established by Associate Professor Adeline Vanderver, a paediatric neurologist at the Children's National Medical Center in Washington DC. The registry collected the medical records and DNA of other undiagnosed Leukodystrophy children and their immediate family, with the intention of grouping like patients into clusters, and then one day performing the exercise Ryan and Stephen had just completed but on cohorts of similar patients. At the time, Stephen had enrolled Massimo on the spot.

'Even back then I was sure there must have been another Massimo out there somewhere.'

Enrolling Massimo in an undiagnosed Leukodystrophies research project proved to have been a prudent step. Stephen contacted Adeline Vanderver and sent her Ryan's extraordinary findings via email. He then followed up with a call to her genetic counselling colleague, Johanna Schmidt. Stephen told her about the interesting finding and of Ryan's incredible dedication and persistence, but soon cut to the chase.

'I have sent Dr Vanderver the report from the familial trio analysis. Could you follow up on the email with her? I was hoping you might have another Massimo.'

He was asking her to review the registry of 800 patients with undiagnosed Leukodystrophies, to find other children similar to Massimo who may be able to back up the DARS finding.

A few minutes later an email arrived that blew the wind back into their sails.

Dear Mr Damiani
Thank you for sharing this information. We have a series of patients with presumed mitochondrial disorders with confluent MRI abnormalities also affecting the corpus callosum/spinal cord similar to what is seen in Massimo. I would be very interested in collaborating with your physicians and would be happy to sequence DARS in these patients, and either provide them with de-identified DNA or the sequence information if we did this here. Please let me know how we can help best explore this exciting new information.
Adeline Vanderver, MD

In a nutshell, Adeline was telling Stephen that she had a group of children who might be potential candidates to validate Ryan's findings of a new disease. After searching through the registry, four patients jumped out as having similar MR imaging and presentation. In fact, she referred to one as a 'dead ringer', with the identical age of onset and progression of symptoms as Massimo. A batch of DNA specimens was sent to Ryan for analysis, with the 'dead ringer' first to be prepared for immediate sequencing and then analysis. No mutations were found in the DARS gene. Stephen's heart sank and for the first time he questioned everything – the feasibility of Mission Massimo altogether, and the decision to put everything in his personal and professional life on hold in order to pursue a diagnosis many suggested was impossible. He even began to doubt his own sanity. But the search continued.

In February 2011, Stephen sent Adeline Vanderver a huge hard drive of genetic data.

'He had mailed us his son's genome,' Vanderver says, with a smile radiating warmth. 'It was the first time a father was ahead of the curve. Up until that moment no layperson I had ever had dealings with was able to dial up to speak our language; it really showed us how much Stephen owned the process.'

Doctors are used to the fact that they usually have to hold a family's hands. 'As scientists and clinicians we are myopic,' she admits. 'When I was in medical school there was this brilliant guy who got a job as a post doc in Italy. At the time, the players in the Italian soccer team had been presented with Maseratis. It was all over the news. We cracked a joke with him that maybe he'd get a Maserati too. We were all floored when he said, "A what?" He was completely oblivious to anything going on around him. As clinicians, we are so used to being the ones to guide our patients along, always in the lead because of our advantage of having greater knowledge about their condition. Too often, though, we aren't good at communicating this information to them. Even my father has spent the last decade not understanding what I do – up until recently, that is.'

Vanderver sees her role now as an interpreter for the science world.

'Stephen had been on our radar for a while, but I didn't realise until that package arrived in the mail just how impressively and rapidly he had retooled himself to such a sophisticated level of scientific knowledge to make this diagnosis happen for his son.'

She remembers the Latin motto of her junior school in Maryland – *Inveniam viam aut faciam* – 'Find a way, or make one.'

'Stephen simply embodied this principle.'

Sally confirms this. 'Stephen is an obsessive details guy – near enough is never good enough. Under no circumstances does he accept the status quo, because in his mind it can always be done better. The best today is not the best tomorrow. When he established Eyre BioBotanics I remember some of the challenges he faced as the first customer for an innovative packaging system he couldn't get working with two of his formulations. There were cheaper and easier alternatives, but he wouldn't accept them because the end result would not be the best finished product. He would obsess for days, adjusting formulations down to three decimal places and fine-tuning manufacturing processes to adjust viscosity, ensuring compatibility at extreme temperatures. He worked through every imaginable scenario in parallel to be certain he could meet a delivery deadline. There must have been a hundred bottles around the house sitting in various incubators and fridges. Eventually it worked, with the end result earning the brand numerous international awards. Stephen is not one to give up once he commits to a goal. My nickname for him is Mr Intensity.'

Adeline Vanderver is a focused person too. She decided at a very early age that she wanted to be a child neurologist.

'My mother tells me that when I was three I insisted on sleeping with a Fisher-Price doctor's bag in which I'd hidden my grandfather's stethoscope, along with some Band-Aids I'd pilfered from the bathroom cabinet. When I was six years old I wrapped my younger sister up, using toilet paper for bandages.'

When she was thirteen, Vanderver read Oliver Sacks' *Seeing Voices*, a book about deaf children. She became fascinated by how language works in the brain. 'We speak not only to tell other people what we think, but to tell ourselves what we think,' writes Sacks. Through her teens, when most of her peers were reading *Cosmopolitan* or *Vogue* magazine, Adeline was devouring everything to do with the subject of neuroscience that she could get her hands on.

'Paediatric neurologists are, on the whole, kind of goofy kids. From an early age I had a passion for all things brain.'

By the time she was at medical school her interest had already begun to focus on unsolved and rare neurological diseases. She went on to specialise in Leukodystrophies.

'It's gruelling work. I often walk around with a stomach ache because I just know I'm missing something. It provokes such deep levels of anxiety for parents not to know the cause of their child's illness. I use all my professional contacts and pull strings endlessly to try to help them. Children with rare diseases, as well as their families, fall through all the cracks of understanding and empathy. When your child is diagnosed with leukaemia, you leave the doctor's office devastated. But you return home to a community (church, school, work, neighbourhood, friends) that understand what this means for your family. They know you will spend months at the hospital, that your child will undergo painful tests and may or may not survive the doctors' efforts to find a cure. They rush to your support and aide – they cook meals, walk your dog and come over just to hold your hand. It's because they know exactly what illness the family are facing.'

By contrast, Vanderver sees what happens to the families of her patients.

'When your child is diagnosed with Leukodystrophy, you leave the doctor's devastated. And you return home to a community that does not understand the desolation created in what you once called your life. They don't understand what lies ahead for you and your child. You are alone.'

This singular difference – this aloneness – is one thing that Vanderver maintains could be changed, even before a cure is found, to improve the life of each and every person with a Leukodystrophy and their family. As a clinician, Vanderver feels this is the biggest gap in advocacy. The thing she most wishes she could change is public understanding of the condition. She points out that even something like muscular dystrophy gets more name recognition, though it is probably no more common statistically.

'Before genomic medicine, the patient and their family were very isolated,' she says. 'Several times a week I get an email from someone out there who has a child with an unsolvable Leukodystrophy. This is all played out in Massimo's story.'

Once the gene thought responsible for Massimo's condition was found, Vanderver started looking at a series of MR imaging scans in other patients. She immediately got in touch with her colleague, Marjo van der Knaap at the VU University Medical Center in Amsterdam, to see if she was keen to work together and have another look at the Myelin Disorders Bioregistry Project patients. Marjo pulled out an additional family that was listed in which two out of the three children were affected. They had information on the parents as well. Adeline had focused on a later-stage abnormality in Massimo's MRI scans, but Marjo reviewed some of the early-stage readings to group them. Marjo's approach made sense genetically because if a pathway is disrupted the onset would be expected to be similar, but not necessarily the final presentation. In early August 2012 the additional families' DNAs were sent to Ryan for sequencing and analysis.

Marjo is a straight talker. She admits Ryan Taft's findings on Massimo didn't interest her much at first.

'To be honest, I wasn't as excited by the report initially as Stephen was. I didn't want to listen because you can't confirm you have discovered a new disease with only one case. You need many patients to prove it.'

The report sat on her desk for months.

'I did nothing with it, until one day my colleague Dr Nicole Wolf told me she had found a new gene for a group of similar patients. It was only then that I saw the connection.'

Nicole knew nothing about Massimo's story, or indeed Ryan's findings of the DARS gene, back in December 2011. In August 2012 she was sequencing the exomes of a small group of patients with imaging reminiscent of LBSL. She assumed these patients would share mutations in a new gene. To her delight, and much to Marjo's surprise, she found mutations in the DARS gene. All of a sudden, there were several more patients with the same condition as Massimo but with a different imaging pattern and clinical presentation. Because of the similarity with LBSL, Nicole and Marjo named the disease Hypomyelination with Brain stem and Spinal cord involvement and Leg spasticity (HBSL).

From there, everything started to fall into place. The hidden language of the children's varied symptoms was finally able to be understood through analysis of their genetic makeup. This isn't a far cry from Marjo's love of classical languages, which she studied as an undergraduate before embarking on the path of medicine.

'I was always a language person. I could have been anything really. There was no specific reason to become a doctor, no grand thoughts of saving lives. I just like to know a lot and I enjoy trying to solve puzzles.'

She went on to study neurology, a specialty she refers to as a 'neat and clear science', and soon became interested in looking at beautiful pictures of the brain through MR imaging. It wasn't until she started working in the field of paediatric neurology that she truly found her passion.

'I really fell for the children. They were so courageous.'

Together with Nicole Wolf and the rest of their team, Marjo van der Knaap was eventually able to identify an entire cohort of children with these two distinct imaging patterns. Sequencing and analysing their exomes over the following month identified mutations in the DARS gene. This all but confirmed the initial diagnosis and the findings were immediately shared with Ryan.

In early September 2012, Ryan received a prestigious UQ Foundation Research Excellence Award in recognition of his work on analysing Massimo's genome. Ryan stood on stage at the awards dinner and gave a brief project overview. At the end of his speech he was surprised to hear

Stephen being called onto the stage. This was Stephen's chance to acknowledge Ryan publicly for all he had done to help Massimo and he wasn't going to miss the opportunity. Two weeks earlier Stephen had had the pleasure of meeting a childhood hero, Apollo 16 Lunar Module Pilot Charlie Duke. Duke was the tenth and youngest person to walk on the moon and was also Capsule Communicator (CAPCOM) for the historic Apollo 11 mission, when Armstrong and Aldrin landed on the surface of the moon. CAPCOM is the vital interface between Mission Control and the astronauts on-board the spacecraft, and Stephen couldn't help but notice a parallel with Ryan's role in Mission Massimo. He told the audience:

> It is the leadership role Ryan has played in linking an international team of clinicians and researchers who have been involved in the common goal of achieving a diagnosis. Beyond Massimo, beyond all of the technology, beyond all of the kilobases and petaflops, Ryan's work offers genuine hope to the many families in the same situation we found ourselves in back in 2009. We may not have the answer just yet, but I am sure we are very close.

Stephen outlined Ryan's extraordinary contribution and spoke of his gratitude to him. He ended his speech by saying:

> On behalf of Massimo I would like to present Ryan with a special gift for all his incredible work – a Mission Massimo plaque. Like all space missions, it has a Mission Massimo

patch, a photo of Commander Massimo 'Mo' Damiani in his NASA space suit signed by Charlie Duke reading 'Reach for the Stars', and Commander Massimo's signature handprint.

The pair embraced on stage in a moving display of patient and research partnership, to great applause. But even on such a special occasion, when Ryan and Stephen sat down it wasn't long before they started to discuss work again, both men well aware that their job was far from over.

They talked about the next steps. Earlier in the day Ryan had received confirmation on the identification of more DARS patients from the Netherlands but couldn't communicate this directly back to Stephen – they had to go through a clinician as it was a research project. If Ryan breached these ethics guidelines he would lose his job. However, he could share general progress – for example that all of the other families from the Myelin Disorders Bioregistry Project had been sequenced. During dinner Stephen promised Ryan that if these families all came back negative he would search the world to find another Massimo and not stop until he did. He knew he would also need to find the funds to sequence them. As he spoke, however, he saw Ryan tense up and Stephen knew he wanted to say something.

'Oh man,' Ryan said. 'This is rough.' Then six words forced themselves out: 'I don't think you need to.'

*

The following week, on 27 September 2012 – 1161 days after Stephen and Sally's world fell apart – Stephen received a phone call. It's a date Stephen and Sally will never forget. Rick Leventer rang mid-morning sounding extremely excited and speaking a lot faster than usual. He enquired if Sally was home to join the call, but she was working from the office that morning. Rick told Stephen he had Ryan on the other line and they needed to talk. Ryan and Rick set up a three-way videoconference and sent Stephen the link to connect. Rick's smiling face appeared on the giant screen on Stephen's desk, then Ryan appeared in another window.

'I could see both of them but I couldn't hear anything. We used sign language to communicate for a couple of minutes as I tried to solve the sound issues. Eventually I ended up dialling in on my mobile and using GoToMeeting for the video. We'd used the bleeding edge of genomic technology to hopefully confirm an unprecedented diagnosis, with a team from around the world, and here we were fumbling to arrange a conference call.'

Eventually, when the technology issues were sorted, Rick opened by asking if Stephen was sitting down before saying there was some news to share and handed over to Ryan. Ryan explained that a family with two affected children had variations in the same gene as Massimo. They had confirmed the diagnosis. Stephen was stunned.

'Wait,' said Rick.

Stephen held his breath, wondering if something was wrong.

'There's more.' Rick was beaming. 'Marjo van der Knaap has identified another group in the Netherlands with variations in the DARS gene.'

'I was completely speechless,' says Stephen. 'I felt the weight of the world lift from my shoulders for the first time in three years. I had placed everything in my life on hold, against the advice of doctors, researchers, family and friends, in order to make this diagnosis happen. I had watched a promising start-up business I'd put so much work into stagnate. As if all that wasn't enough it got slammed by the GFC and the unprecedented increase in the Australian dollar. I had lost contact with so many people because I'd retreated and hid in my study, reading and researching all day and night. I became depressed and relied too heavily on alcohol as a crutch, lost my mojo and felt like I had aged a decade over the previous three years. In May, when the "dead ringer" child's genome had come back negative, I started to question everything – the reality of ever achieving a diagnosis, as well as my own judgement. Who was I to say we're going to get this? On 27 September I had been vindicated for my conviction. I wasn't crazy after all.'

These other children validated Ryan's original finding – they had officially cracked the code. They had successfully identified the cause of a previously unclassified genetic disorder and provided the proof that analysing the trio of parental and child DNA blueprints in parallel – something that had been science fiction when they started this mission in 2009 – provided an effective tool for diagnosing novel and rare genetic disorders. Needless to say, they stunned many in the international medical community.

'It was planned in heaven,' says Marjo.

'Adeline Vanderver was in our sights from very early on,' says Stephen. 'I had read several of her papers which focused on the diagnosis of Leukodystrophies using bio-chemical techniques, molecular genetics and neuroimaging. In establishing the Myelin Disorders Bioregistry Project, she had an "over the horizon" vision of how to poten-tially diagnose these genetically unclassified conditions, well before commercially viable technology existed. She understood that when the cost of whole-genome sequenc-ing came down enough, large cohorts of similar patients enrolled in the bioregistry could have their DNA compared to identify common variations and classify new conditions. Massimo's diagnosis required an international collabora-tion, combining a bottom-up genomic (digital) approach and a top-down clinical and imaging (analogue) approach. If a single member of the team had been removed, we would not be where we are today. The Myelin Disorders Bioregistry Project, however, was a pivotal link in the chain providing the patients who would validate Ryan's finding. Adeline built the ark before the genomic flood, and without it the DARS gene might still be in a bottle floating at sea.'

Adeline Vanderver was thrilled.

'When we asked Ryan to analyse the genomes of more patients in our registry, we immediately found another two who also had the DARS gene defect. Instantaneously, we had a domino effect, with a whole cohort of patients.

And now even more have come out of the woodwork, almost thirty in total. Genomics, coupled with the link-up and collaboration around the world, made this possible. This shrinks the isolation of these families, from Michigan and Colorado to Melbourne.'

Before we look to the future, though, she emphasises that we need to look at the past to see how far genomics has come.

'I've been doing this work for ten years. At first only a handful of diseases was identified, there was a creeping forward in disease discovery. Now it's galloping and diagnoses occur weekly. Of course, the main reason for this is genetic advances, but there are less tangible advances too. I remember back in 2005, my colleague Marjo van der Knaap came to visit from the Netherlands. I would wheel in a huge rolling cart of printouts of MRI scans and pin them up on a white board. It took us three days just to look through all the results. Now, everything is digitised. I can upload the same amount of information on Dropbox and share it with her instantly. These days we spend all our time doing virtual second opinions. Sometimes we can make the diagnosis on image alone. We have quicker diagnoses by virtue of advances in information technology.'

The beauty of studying rare diseases is that they provide a glimpse into the very building blocks of illness. If the faulty gene causing an illness is found, it can lead researchers to identify what has gone wrong with the specific pathway producing essential proteins or chemicals for the body. If they see what happens when one protein is missing then this information can be used to piece together possible causes of more complex and widespread illnesses, such as heart disease, diabetes and cancer.

'It's an astounding technology,' says Vanderver. 'It will completely change medicine the way we know it. It's going to permit not just diagnosis of rare diseases in a more effective way, but will allow us to better understand common diseases. It's likely that many diseases are genetically mediated to some degree, and once we can look at all the genes at the same time we're going to find out that patterns and associations of different changes in various genes can significantly impact your health overall.'

Despite her incredible dedication to her work, Marjo van der Knaap certainly doesn't like being portrayed as a hero.

'We are just doing our jobs,' she says. 'Within five years, we are going to find a diagnosis for all genetic disease and hopefully be able to tailor treatments accordingly. Stephen Damiani was always in the front row, right on top of the quest to diagnose his child's illness. To be honest, I wish there were more like him. Parents are great advocates and we need their incredible energy to push forward this revolution.'

Sally says, 'Stephen called me at work as soon as he got off the phone with Rick and Ryan. I didn't answer initially, as I was in the middle of a meeting with my team. When he kept ringing I thought this must be important, so I kicked them all out and answered the call. To say I was rendered speechless would be an understatement. I wanted to laugh, cry, and jump up and down with excitement all at once. I was trembling for hours and could barely string a sentence together.'

Eager to share the news with the boys' carers, Stephen called Jo and Siobhan, who had taken Massimo, Marco and Leonardo on a cruise along the Yarra River.

'We got it!' he said.

They both screamed with excitement as he explained.

'That night we drank vintage Dom Pérignon,' says Stephen. 'My friend Matt had given us a bottle nine months earlier when we received Ryan's initial report, but we didn't want to open it until the diagnosis was confirmed. It sat next to my desk as a reminder that our mission was not yet accomplished. It was now time to pop the cork.'

At this stage they could only share the news with a small inner circle of family and friends. However, they couldn't resist posting a photo on Facebook of the Dom Pérignon with a cryptic status update reading: 'A very good reason to celebrate!'

Both Stephen and Sally acknowledge that this discovery was significant on many levels. First and foremost, they were no longer alone.

'We now had an army, albeit a small one, to help us in the battle against this disease,' says Sally.

The mystery illness that had struck down her baby son was now a known enemy they could target with a treatment one day.

'We knew what we were dealing with,' she says, 'and the most exciting thing was to learn that some of the patients in the cohort were a lot older than Massimo – teenagers in fact. This meant time might be on our side; we no longer felt that we were racing against a ticking time bomb. Just before we went to bed that evening Stephen asked me if I was okay with the diagnosis. I had no idea why he was asking. Couldn't he tell how over the moon I was, given I had been happily gulping down champagne all evening with him and couldn't wipe the smile off my face for the entire day?

'"Are you comfortable with what we have done with the twins?" he asked.

'Now I understood what he meant. Stephen was checking to see if I was all right with the decision that we had made to have the twins with the help of an egg donor. I have to say, the thought hadn't even crossed my mind. Although I'd had my initial qualms about using a donor when we first set out on our journey, from the moment of their conception it became secondary. I knew as soon as they were born that it wasn't going to be an issue. I felt exactly the same happiness as I did with Massimo.'

Sally thinks about their donor all the time.

'Each night when I tuck the twins into bed, I say a quiet thank you to Melinda. Without her, Stephen and I wouldn't have these wonderful boys in our lives. It's hard to know what life would have been like if we had waited for a diagnosis before contemplating having more children. Would Massimo have blossomed the way he has without his brothers? Would the lightness that entered our home once they were born still have found its way to us without them? And would Stephen and I have maintained the energy to keep pushing for the diagnosis? We will never know the answer to these questions, other than to say that what we did just felt right.'

Now that they had a way to screen her embryos for the gene that affected Massimo, Sally was faced with the option of being able to have another child who would be biologically hers.

'I had absolutely no desire to do such a thing. When Massimo first became ill and we were faced with the prospect of potentially being unable to have more children, I had a definite sense that our family was incomplete. But this disappeared once the twins were born. Five is just the right size. Yes, we took a slightly different road to making it a reality, but we wouldn't have it any other way. If our journey over the past five years has taught us anything, it's that family is not something you take for granted just because you share some genetic material. It is love and understanding between people, the bonds that we form through closeness, through mutual care and respect that matter. Those people I would consider family today are very different from five years ago. Yes, my husband and children, my brother, mother and father feature high on the list, but so too do the carers who have endured our crazy household for so long, when they could have been working a much easier job. And there is our neighbour, Jenna, who is on our doorstep in a heartbeat when I call at 6 am asking for help if Massimo's dressing has come off during the night. It's the friends who haven't been freaked out by a child who can go from squealing in delight one minute to screaming blue murder the next. I may have known this all along, but if it wasn't for one little boy, I may not have realised and appreciated this fact as much as I do today. So, why would I want to change what I have? I often have to pinch myself, to make sure it hasn't all been a dream.'

Chapter 12

WE HAVE HOPE

It took three-and-a-half years to reach the point Stephen and Sally had dreamed of.

'We managed to turn science fiction into science fact,' says Stephen.

They put their tools down and rested for forty-eight hours, but then it was straight back to business. Stephen was not prepared to lose any time.

'Sure, we've cracked the code but now we have to fix it. Achieving the diagnosis was landing Massimo on the moon, an incredible first milestone, but now we must bring him home. We always knew that if we managed to obtain a diagnosis for Massimo, our whole learning curve would start over again and be exponentially more difficult. We'd been so focused on achieving a diagnosis, it was difficult to think beyond it and take in more science. Finding a treatment or cure is an enormous challenge – far more complex and dangerous than the diagnosis and one that has not been successfully achieved before. It's no longer about analysing mountains of data on a computer. The next leaps forward will involve the development and testing of a combination of cellular therapies, which will need direct access to the brain to halt the progression of the disease and repair the damage, and pharmacological compounds. We don't have the luxury of stopping and celebrating our successes either – the clock is still ticking for Massimo and all the other children. There are going to be some tough decisions ahead.'

Stephen's plans to run a marathon had been pushed back because he was so busy, but he started training again after the twins were born and a year later felt fit enough to compete in the upcoming Melbourne Marathon on Sunday, 13 October 2012. The training runs, some as long as three-and-a-half hours, were providing welcome relief from the situation at home. 'As the runs got longer and longer, listening to music began to interfere with my training. I started paying more attention to what my body was telling me. Some say this is the moment you become a runner because you no longer need music as a distraction. Runs became a vital respite for me to clear my head, especially my three-hour runs every Saturday morning. However, after a while the silence began to allow my mind to wander back onto research and stresses at home. I came across audio books and started listening to fiction to give my mind a break from reality. It had been years of relentless research and learning and I needed to just switch off. Home was such a noisy environment with three children and a constant flow of family, therapists, visitors and carers. But what was more distressing was hearing Massimo's constant screams of frustration or pain, especially when he was feeling unwell. It could go on for hours, and it felt like torture to hear him suffering. Although he was always being well cared for, when I was trying to focus on the diagnosis I couldn't block it out because I wanted to help him, and not even noise-cancelling headphones could silence the shrieking. I discovered Matthew Reilly, an incredibly talented action thriller writer, and would look forward as much to hearing the next chapter in the adventures of his Scarecrow and Jack West series as I would to running. I really enjoyed the fresh air as I pounded along the beachfront, my mind focused on the action-packed scenes in an Antarctic ice station or derelict Soviet submarine pen. It would stop my mind wandering back to what was going on at home, providing a brief escape – one that helped to keep me sane and away from the vices that would otherwise have brought me down.'

Despite all of his careful preparations, in early July the Melbourne Marathon had started to look out of reach. Stephen caught a terrible flu that lasted weeks. Then, in late September, he developed pain in his knee, requiring cortisone injections and daily acupuncture.

'The goal of running my first marathon was looking really shaky. On one of my last long runs my left knee failed at 32 kilometres, and I had to catch a taxi home. I was distraught, having trained so hard for so long. With only three weeks to go I wasn't going to make it. We adapted training accordingly and then later in the week I received the call from Rick and Ryan with Massimo's diagnosis. Now nothing was going to stop me. We had achieved the impossible and I was going to run, walk or crawl this marathon, for both me and Massimo.

'On race day I wore a silicone wristband of Massimo's that read "I have something to say". It was how Massimo would indicate he wanted us to get his communication book. I had written in pen on the other side HBSL DARS, and looking down at it made me smile. Nothing was going to stop me, and nothing did for the first 38 kilometres, but then my quads started cramping, soon followed by my hamstrings. I was struggling to walk. I kept looking at Massimo's wristband, though, delirious and laughing at the pain, daring my body to break down now. Four hours and thirty-four minutes after starting, I crossed the finish line, thrilled that I had made it.'

The genetic information about the diagnosis and confirmation of the cause of Massimo's mystery illness was embargoed until the scientific paper had been accepted and gone to press in May 2013. It would be published in *The American Journal of Human Genetics* with the title 'Mutations in DARS cause hypomyelination with brain stem and spinal cord involvement and leg spasticity (HBSL)'. In an almost unprecedented honour, Stephen's name was included as co-author in recognition of his tenacity and involvement as part of the team.

'I may not be medically trained – in fact, I failed a chemistry mid-term in Year 11 – but now I'm published in *The American Journal of Human Genetics*,' he jokes.

As delighted as he was at having achieved a confirmed diagnosis for Massimo, Stephen was also incredibly frustrated. He would have to wait another eight months until the paper was in press and the embargo lifted for him to be allowed to connect with the other families, so that they could share their experiences and all work together to drive and support research into a treatment.

'I was jumping up and down with excitement, wanting to shout from the rooftop, "We've discovered the disease! It's called HBSL and it's caused by a mutation in the DARS gene."'

Adeline Vanderver contacted a colleague at the Children's Hospital Los Angeles with the two patients who had validated the diagnosis. They were the children registered with the Myelin Disorders Bioregistry Project who were selected by Marjo van der Knaap to be sequenced and analysed because their MR imaging at the age of onset was almost identical to Massimo's. Mutations in the DARS gene had lit up like flashing neon lights in both girls' genomes, but Associate Professor Vanderver was unable to tell them what the exact finding was until everything was published. Shortly after the results were officially in print, Stephen and Sally's details were passed on to the family, and the mother of the two girls emailed Stephen:

I can't even begin to find the words to express the wide range of emotions flowing through my body at this time. I have shed many tears . . . just knowing that your family has experienced some of the same feelings of helplessness and wonder concerning what the future holds, as well as the complete desire to defeat the odds. I've often wondered if I would ever meet anyone who could completely understand.

It was incredible for Stephen and Sally to read those words. Soon after, they spoke for three hours by phone, exchanging details and comparing notes about their children's symptoms and the awful struggles they had endured. The family was grateful and overwhelmed at having finally been given a diagnosis for their girls' illness. What was striking for Stephen was how differently the disease had presented in them. The girls, who were six and eleven at the time, were intellectually normal and were verbal with no sign of dysarthria, a motor speech disorder resulting from neurological impairment. When their mother told Stephen that the younger girl had a tethered cord, he nearly fell off his chair. Massimo's tethered spinal cord had always been considered a red herring – an incidental finding that was unlikely to be related to any of his other symptoms. Everything suddenly started to fall into place; this couldn't be a coincidence.

'If there had been a global database of undiagnosed patients, where you could search medical history, symptoms, MR imaging and genomic variations, we may have found a cohort to identify DARS soon after Massimo's initial MRI scan. This is just around the corner now, and highlights the importance of sharing clinical and genetic information.'

When the illness initially presented, the girls had been misdiagnosed with a condition called Acute Disseminated Encephalomyelitis (ADEM) and given a pulse protocol of high-dose intravenous corticosteroids on a monthly basis. This treatment improved their symptoms dramatically and may have influenced their development.

Stephen and Ryan travelled together to the United States in August 2013 to meet the entire family and speak at the Children's Hospital Los Angeles to share the story of how they achieved the diagnosis. At the conclusion of their presentation Stephen made a Skype call to Australia to introduce them to Rick Leventer. Rick initially asked a question through Stephen, who responded by saying, 'Why don't you ask them yourself?' and turned the camera to one of the girls who waved and said hello.

'You could see by the look on Rick's face he was also astonished at the difference in their development compared to Massimo's,' says Stephen.

After all they had gone through over the previous four years, the most crucial breakthrough for Stephen and Sally was this opportunity to connect with other families who had children with mutations in the same gene as Massimo. Now they had two young girls who might give a voice to what it was that Massimo was experiencing.

'It had been so difficult to watch Massimo go through

agonising sensory meltdowns, where he shrieked if there was too much noise or light, ripping wildly at his clothes,' says Sally. 'He endured all that pain and suffering and we had no idea what he was feeling, because he couldn't tell us.'

The girls' mother suggested stripping off Massimo's clothes and moving him to a quiet room at the onset of a sensory meltdown, because her daughters experienced a similarly distressing sensation. They told her that for them it was akin to running nails down a chalkboard resulting in an all-over chilling sensation, paralysing their bodies, which could only be relieved by removing everything in contact with their skin. Since following her advice, Massimo typically calms down within a couple of minutes.

'Beforehand he would scream uncontrollably for up to an hour, becoming violent in a desperate attempt to relieve the sensation, and nothing we tried would ever help. It may seem like a small thing, but this exchange of information inside our little HBSL community has made the world of difference to our lives as a family.'

Back in Melbourne, Stephen suggested to Rick that this early treatment with steroids may have allowed the girls to develop more myelin at a critical stage in the formation of their nervous systems as infants, possibly accounting for their vastly different presentation from Massimo. Previous studies indicated that the DARS gene is preferentially expressed in neuronal or nerve cells, which are the copper wires of the central nervous system. If the neurons were stressed perhaps they were preventing oligodendrocytes – the cells that wrap around them and act as insulation – to form myelin and would respond favourably to corticosteroids. This was not typical of Leukodystrophies, which were considered to be primary white matter disorders.

Rick thought Stephen's suggestion had merit. Corticosteroids sometimes assist with inflammatory neurological conditions, though the improvements are often short-lived and not without serious long-term risks and side effects. 'Massimo is writing his own story and treatment,' he said, 'but I think we should try a high dose of intravenous corticosteroids for a while and see what happens.' They began to trial the treatment on Massimo immediately.

Massimo wasn't the only child to experiment with corticosteroids. In early 2014, Ramakrishna Prasad, the father of Yashovardhan or 'Yasho', a nine-year-old boy from the Netherlands, contacted Stephen and Sally through the Mission Massimo website. Dr Nicole Wolf, Professor van der Knaap's colleague at VU University Medical Center, had diagnosed Yasho with HBSL in the first cohort back in September 2012, and passed on his name. Yasho had just started a pulse protocol of high-dose intravenous corticosteroids and his father was eager to connect with another family, to break their isolation of almost a decade. Early one morning, Stephen was checking emails before the boys woke up and yelled out to Sally: 'Subject 4 has just reached out from the Netherlands – we're going to organise a time to Skype this weekend.'

Again, Yasho's presentation was vastly different from the girls from the West Coast of the United States, and much closer to Massimo's. It was becoming increasingly apparent that the presentation of the disease lay on a broad spectrum of both severity and age of onset, with Massimo the worst affected, the girls least affected and Yasho somewhere in the middle on a scale of severity. Yasho's family spoke to Stephen and Sally again in May, after Massimo had received eight doses of steroids and Yasho was on his third. Massimo was clearly a different child in the second phone call, much happier and more engaged, and Yasho was also showing slight observable improvement in his motor skills and concentration. Now the question was why? Was this possibly due to the steroids having some influence in assisting the growth of myelin? Was there an inflammatory aspect to the disease that the steroids helped settle down? Were some mutations far more damaging than others, or did Massimo have additional mutations in another gene that impacted him more?

No one has answers yet to all these questions, but as more undiagnosed children are sequenced and DARS gene mutations identified as a cause for their mystery illnesses, there will be a greater pool from which to build a natural history for the disease. This will be a crucial step forward for development of a treatment and the move towards a clinical trial.

Recently, Emily Rose, a two-year-old girl from Boston, presented with rapid regression and apparent seizures. The prognosis was bleak and the cause mystifying. One of her medical team, Dr Lance Rodan at the Children's Hospital Boston, came across the HBSL paper published in May 2013 while he was researching the symptoms. He was convinced she had the same condition. DNA from Emily Rose and her parents was sent to VU University in the Netherlands for sequencing of the DARS gene. It identified a compound heterozygous mutation which was the cause of her illness. In just four months, she had received a confirmed diagnosis. The family now have hope, something they could only dream of before. The little girl's mother's thoughts were posted on her Facebook page soon after the diagnosis:

Thank you, everyone, for your thoughts and prayers today. The incredible team at Boston Children's Hospital teamed up with doctors from Massachusetts General Hospital, Australia and the Netherlands to be able to offer Emily Rose some hope for treatment. Further testing is required to determine the best course of action and we will have some hard decisions to make in the next few weeks. However, the overwhelming emotion today is GRATITUDE, because the words 'options' and 'choices' were not even in our vocabulary last week! Again, I am amazed when thinking of the bleak prognosis we were given only four months ago and how far Emily Rose has come . . . can't stop smiling. Hope!!!!

On 16 October 2014, Massimo closed his eyes under general anaesthetic and entered the Siemens MAGNETOM

MRI scanner at the Royal Children's Hospital. It had been twelve months since the first dose of corticosteroids and twenty months since the last MRI scan of his brain and spine.

'Over this period of time we observed significant and sustained behavioural and physical improvements,' says Stephen. 'Massimo is far less irritable, more engaged, and attempts both receptive and expressive communication. His fine motor skills are improved and lower-limb spasticity reduced. Time between the Botox treatments to loosen his calves and hamstrings has been increased from two months to every six months.'

Clinicians and researchers around the world were anxiously awaiting this day, hoping to see an improvement in the MR imaging which reflected improvements in Massimo's clinical presentation. Until now all observations were subjective and, given the uncertainty, it was decided Emily Rose would not start the corticosteroid protocol until Massimo's MR imaging was formally reported. This was judgement day.

The initial local report suggested there were slight changes since the February 2013 MRI scan. However, Stephen requested a copy of the MR imaging on disc so he could immediately FedEx it to Marjo van der Knaap and Nicole Wolf in the Netherlands for their review.

'This wasn't just about Massimo any more. We needed to know if the steroids were working, and confirmation would trigger Emily Rose's doctor to commence her treatment.'

Stephen spent hours poring over the MR imaging with his untrained eyes.

'I could see some subtle changes, but wasn't sure if these were good or bad. However, the images with contrast enhancement and without seemed to look the same where previously there was a difference. I thought this was a positive change, but didn't want to get excited because the last time I thought I saw changes it turned out to be atrophy.'

The following week an email arrived from Marjo van der Knaap and Nicole Wolf, with a report on the MRI. They concluded: 'Compared to the images before starting the treatment this MRI is slightly improved.' Emily Rose was immediately scheduled to commence the same protocol of high-dose intravenous corticosteroids. Within hours of the first infusion her up-pointing toes were relaxed for the first time since she was six months old. Over the following days her uncontrolled eye movements ceased and she was once again able to bear weight through her legs. By Thanksgiving morning she was independently sitting in a high kneeling position for the first time and attempting to pull herself up to stand. She was the fifth child to have shown a favourable response to steroids. 'We stay together, we survive,' says Stephen.

Within two months of the confirmation of Massimo's diagnosis in September 2012, Stephen and Sally were busy establishing the Mission Massimo Foundation to promote the prevention, diagnosis and treatment of childhood

Leukodystrophies. The foundation may carry Massimo's name, but its mission is far broader. It wants to change the economics of rare disease and use HBSL (Condition 0) as proof that we can go from discovering a disease to developing a clinical treatment.

By the end of April 2013, they had obtained all the regulatory approvals and registrations in Australia to act as a non-profit organisation, and soon after started the process in the United States as well to access a far greater pool of philanthropic funding for medical research.

The challenge the foundation faces is that when a disease is perceived as rare the level of attention and funding it receives is almost non-existent. Childhood Leukodystrophies, while individually rare, are not altogether uncommon when including the many misdiagnosed and undiagnosed cases. In fact, childhood Leukodystrophies may affect up to one in 3000 live births, a prevalence not dissimilar to Cystic Fibrosis, yet there are more than 178 open clinical trials for Cystic Fibrosis versus only 16 for childhood Leukodystrophies, of which only five are medical interventions.

'Clearly this is an under served family of conditions. We can't change the rules of the game, but we can change the game itself,' says Stephen. 'If we can reduce the number of undiagnosed cases to less than 10 per cent within five years and, just as we did with the diagnosis, develop a common delivery platform that can treat multiple Leukodystrophies, the game suddenly changes. It will drive public and private investment into research.'

Their strategy is to support early-stage medical research that would otherwise be overlooked, to generate robust supporting data for large government and philanthropic grants.

'It still takes a lot of seed funding to progress this research, and raising public awareness is half the challenge. With so many great causes we needed something truly spectacular to make us stand out. We wanted to pay homage to the Apollo program that had inspired us for Mission Massimo. So, we thought we would try something out of this world. Something like sending someone into space.'

Stephen's idea was to conduct a raffle with a very limited number of tickets for a chance to fly into space. He contacted the two front runners for commercial sub-orbital space travel, Virgin Galactic and XCOR Space Expeditions.

'It didn't work out with Virgin Galactic because of their strict "you buy, you fly" policy, which did not allow tickets to be purchased for competitions. The price of tickets had increased to US$250,000 the week I contacted them, which was a daunting break-even point."'

XCOR was the quiet achiever in commercial space travel. A few hangars down the flight-line from Virgin Galactic at Mojave Air and Space Port, a dedicated group of aerospace engineers pioneered the development of the Lynx – a two-seat re-usable rocket plane using liquid-fuelled re-usable engines. The company didn't have the high profile of its competitor, but it offered a unique flight experience with the passenger sitting in the cockpit.

'In early June I enquired about purchasing a ticket, explaining it was to raise funds for the foundation, and received a response from Astronaut Sales Executive Lara Seveke immediately. A couple of emails and phone calls later we were going to be sending someone into space!'

By August, Stephen had met with representatives of the XCOR Space Expeditions and signed a contract in Los Angeles to send someone on one of the first commercial flights. They would use this as the signature 2014 fundraiser for the Mission Massimo Foundation.

Over the following weeks, foundation board members scrambled to obtain gaming permits and start marketing the raffle to recoup the US$100,000 investment for the ticket and make a profit to fund medical research. On 1 September 2013 the MOMO-001 raffle of 250 tickets at $1000 each was launched. Entrants could purchase tickets for direct entry into the raffle or earn tickets through fundraising in national running events such as Run Melbourne.

'When you reach out to media to raise awareness for childhood Leukodystrophy, the initial response is usually an uninterested "Leukowhat?". When you follow up with "we are sending someone into space" it tends to pique interest pretty quickly. Now we had the fundraising vehicle to grab headlines. The raffle received a full-page write-up in the daily newspaper with a picture of Massimo in a bright-orange space suit holding a model of the XCOR Lynx.'

The foundation would go on to recruit almost fifty athletes for Run Melbourne.

'There was a sea of bright-orange Mission Massimo

Foundation T-shirts at the start line. It was incredibly hard work, but we met our objectives to raise awareness and kick-start vital medical research in our first year. We went from "Leukowhat?" to front-page news, raising the profile of childhood Leukodystrophy beyond our wildest expectations,' says Sally.

When Stephen visited XCOR Space Expeditions in Mojave California to present them with a plaque in appreciation of their support, he was allowed inside a spacecraft. 'As you might imagine I was pretty excited to be able to do that. Most of all, I was thrilled to share how an adventure to the stars was powering a mission far beyond.'

With the funds raised from the successful MOMO-001 raffle and generous philanthropic contributions, the Mission Massimo Foundation launched its Joint Strike Vector research project to develop a common gene therapy platform for the treatment of multiple childhood Leukodystrophies. Testing is scheduled to commence on preclinical models in 2015.

One of the most experienced gene therapy researchers for neurological conditions in the world now lives in Australia. Associate Professor Matthias Klugmann used to be laboratory head at the universities of Heidelberg and Mainz, and became a partner of LeukoTreat, a project funded by the European Commission aimed at developing therapeutic strategies for a large number of Leukodystrophy-affected patients. In 2010, he was made head of the Functional Genomics Group in the Translational Neuroscience Facility at the University of New South Wales, and was awarded a prestigious Future Fellowship by the Australian Research Council for his research program on metabolic changes in Leukodystrophies.

When Professor Klugmann was in Melbourne for a conference, Stephen seized the opportunity to meet him. 'This was our chance to take a disease that had only been confirmed four weeks earlier, right up to the front of the queue for developing a clinical treatment.'

Gene therapy is an experimental technique that essentially uses corrected or healthy DNA as a drug to treat disease. The most common form of gene therapy involves the use of a vector to transport a healthy copy of the broken gene into target cells. There is hope that in the near future, clinicians will be able to treat many genetic disorders in this way.

'In theory, we can use a virus to carry a working copy of the DARS gene into cells where it is broken,' says Stephen. 'This may prevent the condition progressing further and maybe even allow for the formation of new myelin. Ideally, gene therapies, once further developed and proven for safety and efficacy, could be given before a child shows symptoms, to prevent the onset of the disease altogether. Recent human clinical trials using Adeno-Associated Viruses (AAV) for gene therapy in Canavan Disease have shown great promise, and Matthias was involved in this work. The technology is not quite there yet, but once it is, and I don't think we are that far off, it will further support the case for expanded newborn screening. In its ultimate form, the technology may one day provide genetic immunisation against life-threatening conditions, where early intervention is critical.'

Back in early 2013, Ryan Taft was already looking at the first steps on how to model and potentially treat Massimo's condition using stem cells. Ryan had contacted a colleague at the University of Queensland's Australian Institute for Bioengineering and Nanotechnology (AIBN), Associate Professor Ernst Wolvetang. His laboratory uses stem cells that are 'pluripotent' as disease models, meaning they can differentiate into any adult cell type and therefore have tremendous potential for individualised disease therapy.

Using some of Massimo's skin cells – called fibroblasts – Ernst created a line of stem cells and then differentiated them into neuronal precursor cells, the type of nervous tissue that makes up the basic wiring of the human brain. The results were striking. After six days growing in a Petri dish in the lab, the cells were extremely stressed compared to a control line of normal cells without DARS mutations. The division cycle for these cells consists of four discrete phases: M, G1, S and G2. Massimo's stem cells displayed a prolonged G1 phase and reduced S phase, the critical point when DNA replication occurs. The DARS gene encodes for an enzyme in humans called Aspartyl-tRNA synthetase. In an experiment introducing excess aspartic acid to the growth medium of the stem cells, the cell cycle showed partial recovery. This would suggest that there may be a potential therapeutic benefit from supplementation with aspartic acid. However, the dosage levels need to be carefully set as excess aspartic acid may be toxic and potentially even lethal. Specialists are now working to create the right aspartic acid supplementation protocol for clinical trial in 2015, which Stephen has nicknamed 'Massimo's Moondust'.

'The next step will be to create a line of stem cells from Massimo, with the DARS mutations corrected using a new genetic editing technology known as CRISPR (Clustered Regularly Interspaced Short Palindromic Repeats), which makes specific changes in the DNA sequence,' says Stephen. 'One day we may be able to implant these corrected cells to repair damage caused by the condition without the risk of rejection, as they are his own cells.'

When Stephen and Sally visited the AIBN to thank Ernst and update him on the fundraising, they had their first chance to see Massimo's cells under a microscope.

'It's strange to see your son's brain effectively growing in a Petri dish, but incredibly exciting. We have some of the best and brightest minds in the world leading this cutting-edge research right here in Australia, and we want to do everything possible to support them. In the tradition of having an Apollo-style mission patch for all our research, we are calling this one the Prometheus project, after the film *Prometheus* in which humanity's forerunner, the "Engineers", tweaked human DNA,' says Stephen.

In order to test these therapeutic interventions beyond the Petri dish and push towards human trials, a preclinical mouse model is required. Since 2011, when Stephen and Ryan considered creating a genetically engineered mouse model to validate the DARS finding, the cost has come down dramatically, with the availability of CRISPR technology. Rather than spending two years or longer going through multiple generations to make a mouse model, with CRISPR it is now possible to generate a genetically engineered mouse in one step within weeks. On 22 July 2014, the same day Massimo turned six, Dr Marco Herold from the Walter and Eliza Hall Institute of Medical Research commenced work on the MASSIMOUSE – a CRISPR mouse model of HBSL.

Colonel Chris Hadfield, a Canadian astronaut, says you can't live a worthwhile life without taking risks – it is only in this way that dreams and fantasies are turned into reality. He reflects on his time as commander of the International Space Station: 'You have the opportunity to go around the world every ninety minutes with the view of Earth from your window. All you have to do is flip yourself upside down and suddenly the rest of the universe is right there at your feet.'

Turning things on their head is exactly what Stephen Damiani did to diagnose his son. In the space of only five years Stephen and Sally went from being faced with a mystery illness that was going to claim their son, to the diagnosis of a new disease. Since then researchers have already made significant in-roads to understanding HBSL, and hope to advance to using cellular therapies in human clinical trials. It is still early days but if these efforts are successful, just as with the diagnosis, they hope to adapt the cellular therapy platforms to treat other genetic conditions and change the economics of rare disease altogether. In the medical world, the pace of their progress is extraordinary. For Stephen Damiani, though, whose little boy's life depends on finding a treatment now, it's not fast enough.

Stephen reflects on what drove him to look so determinedly for a diagnosis for his son. He admits that, more than anything, it was the crippling fear that one day Massimo would outlive him and be unable to care for himself.

'I couldn't imagine leaving him with no one around to care for him unconditionally like we do as his family.'

When Massimo was first diagnosed and was deteriorating so rapidly, Sally was constantly anxious about how much time they would have left with him and what would happen when he died.

'Would we be in hospital or at home? Would we be holding him when it happened? The same thoughts would cycle through my head, especially in the still of the night when I would be rocking Massimo back to sleep. During those moments there was nothing else to distract me. Initially, he lost such major skills – standing, sitting, walking, talking – but once his regression stabilised, the changes were far more subtle. Even so, those horrid thoughts of losing Massimo still occupied a space in my mind, albeit a much smaller one. Soon they started to be replaced with wondering what would happen to Massimo when we go.'

Sally and Stephen can't imagine Massimo living

anywhere but in their house, under their care. The load is shared with a small group of people, including Sally's mother, their carer of more than four years, Siobhan, and his loving godmother, Jo – Team Massimo as they like to call it.

While Massimo is generally a good-natured little boy, who is usually smiling and very affectionate, he does suffer from a sensory processing disorder, a common condition for children with disabilities. This means he has difficulty interpreting and regulating external stimuli.

'Sometimes Massimo just gets overloaded, and cannot tolerate any new sensory input,' says Sally. 'When this happens we turn off the lights and television, remove all his clothes and give him an icepack to play with until he calms down. Everyone knows the drill now when he starts – and by "start" I mean Massimo will scream uncontrollably. The twins are chaperoned out of the room, and he usually starts to calm down after a few minutes. I can see that if a stranger walked into our home as all of this was unfolding, they might think it was a bit weird. And I wonder how this would be handled if Massimo was in an institution. Would he be doped to a point where this no longer happened, to make him easier to manage?'

Massimo is relatively small for six years. While he is still young, Sally and Stephen can lift him to move him from his wheelchair to his stroller, as well as to get him in and out of bed, the car and the shower.

'He is getting heavier but in some ways it's like having a really big baby,' says Sally. 'I know it's going to get harder as he grows. Life will be more restrictive, but we'll just work with it; we certainly won't be the first ones to have to deal with that. I do wonder, though, whether some of the things he does now, such as crawling around the house, or chewing on anything he can get his hands on, will seem out of place when he's a teenager growing stubble on his chin. And whether the little gurgling sounds he makes instead of being able to talk will still sound cute when his voice breaks.'

Sally feels that Massimo's physical limitations are the easiest to deal with in many ways. The greatest challenge is Massimo's lack of verbal communication, which is not only a source of frustration, especially for him, but also makes it hard for them to ascertain his cognitive abilities.

'If we could give Massimo one skill back, it would be his ability to speak. At least that would allow him to tell us what he needs.'

When he turned five, Massimo was assessed by neuropsychologists as having the mental capacity of a child of twelve to eighteen months.

'He still enjoys watching *Baby Einstein*, which is meant for nine- to eighteen-month-old babies,' says Sally. 'I always feel conflicted playing this for him. It's so obvious when you see his eyes light up that he loves the show, but I always wonder if I should force him to watch something other six-year-olds would enjoy, or is it mean to deprive him of his small pleasures?'

Sally finds beauty and joy in the sheer fact that Massimo is alive, rather than in the small achievements he notches up. Both she and Stephen focus on reinforcing his current skills, even though they hope one day these will improve. Nonetheless, her fears for his future run deep, sometimes overshadowing her optimism.

'The thought of Massimo being cared for by others because Stephen and I are no longer around is petrifying,' she says. 'Especially given he cannot talk.'

She is referring to reports that are regularly in the media about disabled adults being sexually and physically assaulted in homes.

'I feel ill each time I read one of those articles and often find myself crying uncontrollably. I clearly remember a morning when I shared an article with Stephen and he became even more determined to push for a diagnosis, making a promise that Massimo would never need to be institutionalised. He says those articles sit in the back of his mind as a constant reminder of the potential conse-quence of failure.

'I don't think that we will ever shake this fear of Massimo living in a world without Stephen and me being there to care for him. It will remain unless we find a cure.' Sally accepts that they cannot live in the grip of this fear forever and that the problem of adequate housing and care for the disabled is an issue that she will need to tackle in the future. 'For now, we are throwing all of our energy behind finding a treatment for Massimo and helping him to develop as much as possible with the supportive thera-pies we have in place today.'

While they hope they will be able to develop a treatment

for Massimo that makes this problem redundant, they are also realistic about if and when that might happen.

'Even though achieving the diagnosis was an incredible milestone, it was fundamentally a computational biology problem,' says Stephen. 'Now we are dealing with some far greater challenges, such as crossing the blood–brain barrier and targeted gene delivery. We are buoyed by the fact that there have recently been major advances in gene and stem-cell therapies. These experimental treatments have typically prevented the onset of a condition, or slowed its progression in some cases. However, none have successfully repaired damage caused by a breakdown of myelin. We can only hope these breakthroughs happen in time to make a difference to Massimo.'

Chapter 13

THE MASSIMO EFFECT

Disease has no regard for timing, no respect for age. Disease is impatient and ruthless, not even waiting for an infant's first breath before overtaking its tiny body floating inside the protective armour of its mother's womb. Disease weaves its way into every cell, into the very alphabet of life; four proteins twisted together like coloured beads on a child's bracelet – ATCG, TACG, CATG – already forming the blueprint of who we will become once we are born.

Conquering disease has been the goal of the medical profession, and antibiotics one of its greatest weapons. But medicine is in the throes of a quiet revolution. Many experts maintain that we are already well on our way to a cure for a host of genetic illnesses and cancers, with the possibility of tailor-made medication for each and every patient from the comfort of the doctor's desk at the local clinic.

'The future has arrived,' says Ryan Taft. 'Children are now being diagnosed every day using whole-genome sequencing. Massimo opened up the floodgates. We were the first in the world to discover a new genetic disease by sequencing a child and both his parents and then analysing the data from this trio. Once we knew we had solved Massimo's case, we had a system in place that could be applied to other children. But that's where the story begins, not ends.'

Ryan and Stephen are modest men who shirk the limelight. In diagnosing Massimo, they created the blueprint for diagnosing genetic diseases of all kinds. And the team of researchers and clinicians they collaborated with from around the world laud the pair's achievement. Every diagnosis paves the way for another.

'We have come to call this the Massimo Effect,' says Ryan. 'The direct knock-on effect of Massimo was the diagnosis of more than 100 children in less than two years, with an incredible range of illnesses, from epilepsy to cognitive brain disorders. We have also identified some new disease-causing genes we never knew existed.'

And there will be many more to come. Sydney girl Mielle Dale is an example. In 2012, at the age of four, she showed rapid deterioration in both speech and balance. MR imaging was compatible with a condition called Leigh Syndrome, a potentially fatal disease that reduces the ability of the mitochondria, the powerhouses of the body's cells, to produce energy. A pharmaceutical company in the United States was conducting a clinical trial of a new drug for Leigh Syndrome and all ten children enrolled showed marked improvement in their symptoms. However, without a definitive genetic diagnosis, Mielle was not eligible to participate. The six family members were sequenced in less than two weeks, and within a month a previously unknown mitochondrial gene mutation was identified. Mielle was immediately admitted into the clinical trial and she is showing a tremendous response to the experimental therapy.

'What started out as a project we pieced together with duct tape and baling wire, became more than we could ever dream of,' says Ryan.

Particularly rewarding for Ryan was the collaborative nature of the international group that worked on diagnosing Massimo.

'I wasn't just seen as a lab rat – I was part of a multi-disciplinary team.'

Ryan Taft's career has taken him on a trajectory he could not possibly have imagined back in 2010. He has shot from young bench scientist, to Director of Scientific Research at Illumina, notching up some remarkable achievements along the way. What's next on his agenda?

'Let's do all the kids who have debilitating rare diseases now, using genomics,' he says quietly, with a smile on his face. 'I would hope that when a child is suspected of having a Leukodystrophy, we would use MR imaging and clinical presentation, together with mapping their genome to rapidly give us the diagnosis. It's a moral imperative. I'd like to see the terrible diagnostic odyssey families still have to endure completely evaporate, and I think there's a good chance that's going to happen within the next few years. What we did in Massimo's case was definitely a peek into the future. What does the world of medicine look like when no one with a genetic disease goes undiagnosed? What happened with Massimo will be happening with everyone across the globe eventually; it's the whole gambit, the future of medicine. If your father has a heart attack you will be able to see if you carry the same gene that influenced his heart disease in the first place. This is truly personalised medicine. I would hope it won't be too long before we see this kind of technology inside the doctor's clinic, sitting right there on the desk.'

Illumina recently hired Ryan to help with braiding both genetic and clinical information together to achieve diagnoses. At the age of thirty-six, it's his first time in eighteen years away from the bench, wearing a suit instead of a white lab coat. In April 2014, he and his heavily pregnant wife, Erica, together with their two-year-old daughter, Rowan, packed up and moved back to Ryan's home town of San Diego in California, where Illumina is based, to take up his new position.

What was so special about what Ryan, Stephen and the team achieved with Massimo?

'It wasn't just the outcome that was incredible,' says Stephen. 'It was the fact we were first and did it all on a shoestring.'

'The bench guy and the dad drove the show,' Ryan agrees. 'It was the sheer dogged determination of all the people involved at the vanguard that helped tip the pyramid upside down in the medical world.'

People ask Ryan why he is focusing so much of his attention on rare childhood diseases.

'If we are truly looking to the future we need to start with rare genetic disorders. Refining our tools on this as a control population is a solid foundation – then we can go on to tackle more complex diseases caused by more than one isolated gene. We are planting seeds now that are going to tell our genetic story in the future.'

Rick Leventer says of Ryan: 'The guy's unique. His willingness to take this project on was truly extraordinary. Together, Stephen and Ryan have been the first to build a template for diagnosing genetic diseases that others can now use. They led the pack.'

Stephen hopes that beyond Massimo, collective efforts will pave the way to diagnose many other children and perhaps even cure their rare genetic disorders in the future.

'Nowadays, there is no technical reason why a newborn can't have their whole genome sequenced to identify many life-threatening diseases in less than twenty-four hours. Within several years it may even be possible to genetically immunise against some conditions detected through newborn screening and prevent the onset altogether. Above all, this new approach to medicine offers hope to the many families who find themselves in the terrible situation we were once in ourselves.'

Stephen believes many new innovations in health and wellbeing will be driven by patients, who need to start being viewed as consumers. He envisages that the first to take on this new technology will be the 'worried wealthy', to be followed within five years by the mass 'clinical consumer'.

'History has shown that the fortunate and privileged are the ones who have been able to access new technology first and drive costs down through increasing volume. They are the early adopters, the innovators, driving the take-up of inventions into the mainstream. We've seen this happen with ocean liners; aviation; hybrid, electric and fuel-cell cars and now even commercial sub-orbital space travel. The same diffusion of innovation is going to be seen with personalised health and wellbeing, powered by genomics.'

'It is a complex area and brave new ground for all involved,' says Ryan. 'Although in this new age of genomic medicine we are getting better at finding mutations, it's still a huge leap to translate these discoveries into specific treatment, especially when it comes to a newly recognised genetic disorder in a gene like DARS, the one we found responsible for Massimo's disease, that has previously not been described as being associated with any disease.'

What do you do with potential findings that are unrelated to the focus of the search, caught up in the drift net as you trawl through masses of information? The ethical considerations raised by genome sequencing are enormous. One of the pitfalls of sequencing and analysing a child's entire DNA is that researchers may find aberrations leading to conditions that only become evident later in life. For example, would a parent want to know that their child carries a gene that increases the risk of Alzheimer's as they age? And what about the child's rights?

'As scientists in the lab, we don't look at these incidental findings,' says Ryan, 'but it becomes a thornier issue when rolled out in the clinic. For example, how do we deal with insurance companies who may look at the genetic readout of a potential client and refuse to insure them? There is a revolution on our doorstep and most people don't even know about it.'

'Massimo is a beacon for what is going to come,' says Dr Bartha Maria Knoppers, Director of the Centre of Genomics and Policy in the Faculty of Medicine at McGill University in Montreal.

'We are seeing not just the impact of whole-genome sequencing, but also the rebirth of interest in rare diseases. This has been brewing for the past few years. We have traditionally thrown lots of money into research around common diseases, such as obesity, effects of alcohol and smoking, but this is changing.'

She explains that having a rare disease is akin to being in no-man's-land. Now we have a quicker way to name a disorder. The new technology is not only helpful in the diagnosis and treatment arena, it is important in the realm of prevention of disease. The problem as she sees it lies with what we do with incidental findings.

'There is a twist in all this that's unique to paedi-atric patients. They present us with a challenging ethical scenario. As adults, we have a choice as to whether or not we want to know our genetic blueprint. In Canada, legislation determines that parents of a minor may opt out of being told of any incidental genetic information garnered through genome sequencing. It is their right not to know. The exception is where something clinically significant is found that is actionable and preventable, which will become apparent in childhood. In that case, the parents will be informed of those conditions.'

She believes the medical profession's paternalistic musings are being challenged like never before. There are, of course, traditional pitfalls, such as how much we actually understand about risk and susceptibility.

'Risk is such a subjective and personal factor. I don't think we've quite figured it out yet. Our choices are affected culturally too; they are dependent on context, socioeconomic factors and religious beliefs.'

In the near future, Dr Knoppers believes people will have to consent to what they *don't* want to know. It's the reverse of informed consent. She maintains we are going to have to re-educate our general practitioners who are currently not trained in genomic medicine.

'We need stories like Massimo's,' she says. 'The more stories we hear about young researchers who spend their free time passionately following what interests them rather than just being on the treadmill to publication – who truly connect to a particular family or individual – the better. They make it their personal quest. Knowledge goes past the data when you engage with communities. The more people involved, the more it will inspire and give the researcher hope. It's like having an enthusiastic cheer squad behind you. The human side of research should never be lost to young researchers; this keeps them ambitious, without needing to be cut-throat.'

Both Adeline Vanderver and Rick Leventer acknowledge they would never have reached a diagnosis if they had no other option than to keep working solely at trying to piece together answers from Massimo's symptoms and MR imaging alone. Vanderver sees genomics becoming a tornado in the medical world today.

Professor John Mattick, Ryan Taft's mentor when he was still a lab scientist at the Institute for Molecular Bioscience in Queensland, now heads up the prestigious Garvan Institute of Medical Research, one of only three institutions in the world to house the latest next-generation DNA sequencing machine – the Illumina X Ten. His vision is for the Garvan Institute to be one of the top facilities in the world overseeing the entire process of diagnosing rare diseases. By combining sequencing and bioinformatics with interpretation, it would make it a clinical reality for every family in a similar circumstance to Massimo's family to obtain a diagnosis for their child in the future.

'There have been three revolutions in genetics,' says Professor Mattick. 'Discovering the double helix structure of DNA allowed us to see what a gene looks like. Then came cloning, which provided us with a window into gene complexity. Now we have genomics – an unrecognised seismic shift in the medical world.'

What Ryan Taft and Stephen Damiani did with Massimo, according to Professor Mattick, is like a preview of what will affect all of our lives in the not too distant future.

'We will all be having our genomes mapped soon. Personalised medicine is a revolution that is already upon us and genomics is going to be everywhere we can possibly imagine. Massimo is at the vanguard of this movement, and his father, Stephen, is a leader of the trend. He sees that we are turning medicine from being the art of crisis management into the science of good health. Forewarned is forearmed.'

'We are certainly at the tipping point,' says Ryan Taft's former lab colleague Professor Marcel Dinger, who is now Head of Kinghorn Centre for Clinical Genomics at the Garvan Institute. He is happy to press the send button on his iPad and forward a copy of his personal genome, excited to share the vital and personal information it holds. 'We need a global alliance. What people don't understand is that the more genomes we map, the bigger the database we can extract useful information from. The broad sharing of information is crucial in helping us diagnose and treat not only rare diseases, but also illnesses such as cancer and heart disease.'

The Garvan Institute's five-year goal is to develop a routine, simple diagnostic test for rare and inherited diseases, using next-generation sequencing technology. Part of this project will be to characterise the development of cancerous tumours and apply similar techniques to pharmacogenomics – the study of how genes affect an individual's response to specific medications – for a tailored or individualised approach to prescribing.

'Stephen Damiani's drive is extraordinary,' says Professor Dinger. 'He pushed this research well before any of the clinicians. Stephen solved his son's unknown genetic disorder way ahead of the curve. At the time, it was done through sheer determination and a little serendipity. The Garvan Institute is busy trying to put infrastructure into that process.'

Speaking at the Illumina Understand Your Genome conference recently, hosted at the Garvan Institute, Stephen shared the story of his family's journey and how it provides a real insight into the impact of genomics. As part of the conference he took the opportunity to have his own genome re-sequenced and loaded into the Understand Your Genome application on an iPad.

'Up until that point, copies of my genome were sitting on various hard drives in the bottom drawer of my desk, as well as at several research institutes around the world. The data had never been analysed other than to diagnose Massimo, but I always wanted to unlock the information it contained about my own health and this was a great opportunity.'

It showed he is a carrier for two conditions and is predisposed to a common blood clotting disorder, as well as a condition that increases his risk of developing a benign growth on the pituitary gland. Stephen wants to maximise his health so he can be around a long time to watch over his three sons and drive forward research. He has already taken pre-emptive steps in the light of these findings. He takes aspirin daily and wears compression stockings on long-haul flights. In addition, he has undergone screening for any pituitary growths, through a series of blood tests and a brain MRI. Even though there is a 30 per cent lifetime risk of a benign tumour developing, he will be routinely monitored to ensure early intervention should a growth develop.

'There are many things that influence our wellbeing. Genetic information is just one valuable data source able to help me make informed decisions about my health. I am well aware the mirror and my belt buckle are equally as important, probably more insightful and less ambiguous.'

Stephen is challenging essential questions about accessing this new technology.

'I'm allowed to walk out this door, drink myself stupid, smoke and eat junk food, all of which have known serious health impacts, but I am restricted in seeking genetic information about myself to make decisions that may prevent the onset of disease or improve my wellbeing and lifestyle. Admittedly, on the flip side, I may also learn about diseases with no interventions. Even so, no one has the right to prohibit me from accessing my own genetic data. I am opting to find out this information and I am informed enough about the concurrent risks to provide valid consent.'

Stephen is somewhat perplexed by public angst over the sharing of genetic information. 'Unlocking and sharing this information is vital to identifying genetic variations which cause or influence many diseases. The more data we have, the greater confidence we acquire, allowing more precise lifestyle choices and ultimately the development of targeted therapies.' He does concede that there is a potential danger that the information can be used against you, and this demands ongoing public discussion to ensure the regulatory frameworks are in place to protect individuals from any form of discrimination. He firmly believes it should be unlawful to discriminate against any individual in any way simply because of their genetic makeup.

'We already know an individual is not the sum total of their DNA; environmental factors have a huge influence as well. If we take a big-picture, long-term view of the issue,' says Stephen, 'it is actually in the best economic interest of health systems and insurance companies to support the genomic transformation of medicine, and provide preventive options for good health. After all, you have to be alive to pay your premiums.'

The hysteria surrounding genomics reminds Stephen of where we were back in the mid-1990s with the advent of e-commerce.

'People were afraid their credit-card number would be stolen, but at the same time were happy to hand their card over to some random waiter at a corner restaurant who could just as easily jot down all the private details. Twenty years later, e-commerce has changed the way we live, overwhelmingly for the better.'

Stephen points out that more genetic data will likely be

generated over the next six months than will have been generated throughout history. Sequencing is now the commodity, as he sees it. The challenges are in the inter-pretation and communication of this information.

'The traditional one-hour face-to-face consult will not be able to support the genomic revolution – it's going to require a radically different e-health model.'

'The future of genomics is full of promise, but there are still issues to be resolved,' agrees Ryan Taft. 'There has been an explosion in personalised medicine. Current genetic testing is faster and cheaper and will soon replace old diagnostic protocols. We are looking at the structure of the genome and testing drugs using this technology that will work for the individual. In principle, a private hospital can already sequence every newborn in their labour ward, with a view to prevention and tailored treatment from the beginning of a person's life. What concerns me most is that the public doesn't understand this is happening.'

How do you start to lock this down, protecting the rights of individuals to the privacy of their own, or their child's, genome?

'The horse left the barn a long time ago,' Ryan says. 'We need more public discussion about genomics and its impacts. It's going to affect everyone. The technology is out there and both public institutions and private companies are already using it. We need to ensure data security – how do you maintain your genome in a safe place, for example? Do you carry it around with you on a chip attached to your key ring? The cost has come down from $2.7 billion for the first complete genome in April 2003, which took thirteen years to sequence – to, in theory, your genome being sequenced in twenty-four hours for $1000. Currently most clinicians use MR imaging for diagnosis, which costs around $1500. Within eighteen months to two years they will almost certainly be looking at a patient's genome as well.'

Medicine traditionally takes the historical approach. It focuses on diagnosis through symptoms and then bases the treatment on that; it's primarily reactive. This is being turned on its head, as the genomic revolution allows the prevention and management of many conditions through its genetics. Stephen saw this early on during Massimo's diagnostic odyssey: 'Medicine is going from an analogue to a digital model, but there is an important overlap. In order to diagnose Massimo, we needed to marry his clinical analogue presentation (phenotype) with its genetic digital cause (genotype). You can't work with either in isolation.'

He strongly believes that genomic sequencing is just another tool in the medical toolbox, albeit a powerful one.

'You can put all the ingredients for the perfect meal into a Thermomix, but it will never taste the same as one that's been made with love. That X-factor judgement made possible by the human mind will never be completely replaced by 1's and 0's.'

The true economic cost of diagnosing Massimo was close to a million dollars; sequencing was only a small fraction of the total amount. But how do you put a figure on the huge toll taken on the mental and physical health of the Damiani family?

'I'm sure it took more than a few years off my life. But who knows, perhaps I can get them back through looking at my genome now. Would I rather have an undiagnosed child and be living in purgatory without hope? Absolutely not. Without all this we wouldn't have had Leonardo and Marco, who have shown us the true meaning of family. When I learn another child has been diagnosed or a new condition has been discovered using the blueprint developed for Massimo, well, that doesn't have a price. I still pinch myself that we played a part in an incredible team of dedicated clinicians and researchers who achieved the impossible. Most of all I'm proud of Massimo for being the catalyst that made it all possible.'

'*Everything happens for a reason,* sounds like such an innocuous phrase,' says Sally. 'I am the first to throw it around when a friend has ended a long-term relationship, or if someone suddenly loses a job.'

When Massimo became ill, Sally was at a loss to understand why it happened.

'Why does any child have to get sick, really? Unfortunately, when you live in the world of disability and childhood illness, you often meet people whose children die at a young age. Sometimes, they are comforted by the thought that their children are little angels, destined for greater things. Personally, I am still at odds with how one reconciles terminal disease with young innocent children – it just seems infinitely unfair.'

Stephen's trainer, Brian Rabinowitz, who took on the role of mentor as well as fitness coach, once said that Massimo had chosen his parents. Sally wonders if it was destiny that Massimo would be born into their family and become the inspiration for a potential revolution in medicine.

One night, Sally and her brother went out for dinner together, a rare event. John told her he believed that finding Massimo's diagnosis was Stephen's calling in life.

'Stephen is not going to be remembered for skin care,' he said. 'He will be remembered for diagnosing and fixing Massimo.'

Both Sally and Stephen are struck by many little coincidences that have occurred along the way. From Sally meeting Leah for the first time when she came into the clinic when Leah's colleague was off sick, to the nurse who ushered Leonardo into his life-saving cardio surgery being so similar to Melinda, their egg donor. Then there was Leah's off-the-cuff remark about bioinformatics and genetics to Erica over a casual cup of coffee, which ended up being a key to the chain of events that led to the unlocking of Massimo's diagnosis. They wonder if these were all signs that there were greater forces at play.

'When we think about how this all came together,' says Sally, 'I think serendipity played a vital part in the equation. After everything that has happened to us, I am very tempted to believe *everything happens for a reason*.'

Ryan Taft is a man of science and doesn't hold much faith in destiny; he proudly wears a T-shirt his wife, Erica, bought him, emblazoned with the words *Show Me the Data*. What he does believe strongly, though, is that the events leading up to Massimo's diagnosis have had serious knock-on effects in the clinical adoption of the technology.

'It happened in everyone's backyard, right here in Australia. I don't think it will be too long before this is an everyday occurrence. The conversation around genomics is evolving so quickly.'

At a Key Opinion Leaders' summit in San Diego at the end of 2014, Dr Howard Jacob, Director of Human and Molecular Genetics Center at the Medical College of Wisconsin, told a packed room: 'I can think of no other diagnostic thing we can do in medicine that has such enormous benefit from the day you are born until the day you die.'

Massimo's seventh birthday is now fast approaching, and everyone is amazed at how far he has come since the awful events surrounding his first birthday. Despite the forthcoming celebrations, it is still a deeply emotional time for Sally and Stephen.

'His birthday marks the anniversary of the identification of Massimo's Leukodystrophy,' says Sally, 'and it's hard not to think about where Massimo may have been if he hadn't fallen ill. We're grateful for all his achievements, though – it's hard to believe he's finished his first year of school. He's really a different child from what he was twelve months ago, before he started the steroid treatment. Overall he's calmer, stronger, far more engaged and interacts happily with other children. The other day he even said "Mum".'

In a photo taken recently at a friend's birthday party, Massimo is seated between his brothers on an ordinary small red chair, his eyes focused on a plate of food.

'We could see how much his fine motor skills have improved,' says Stephen. 'He must have eaten his body weight in French fries.'

Sally laughs. 'Later on, when he was back in his wheelchair, Massimo suddenly noticed the jumping castle. He was like a man on a mission. He zoomed over by himself and the second I unstrapped him he rushed inside to join in the fun. He's really developing his own little personality.'

Sally and Stephen are now determined to bring some normality back into their lives, after nearly six years of the relentless search for answers to their son's mystery illness.

'We became social recluses during that time,' says Stephen. 'It was hard not to feel guilty going out when we could have been at home working on how to fix Massimo. All those years we barely had a break, so now we are trying to spend weekends together as a family, having fun with our kids.'

Stephen has set his sights on running another marathon in 2015, recognising how easily he falls back into bad habits if he doesn't focus on his health and fitness. He's set himself a goal to run a marathon in each home town of the other HBSL children in 2016/2017. Meanwhile, Sally has taken on a new role at work, in a different company that has a great team environment. Thankfully, she is finding it increasingly easy to balance home life and work, and hopes to join Stephen for her first marathon soon.

'It still feels like we are walking a tightrope sometimes, but we don't fall off as much as we used to,' says Sally.

Finding the specific gene responsible for his son's illness was the only hope Stephen had of understanding what the future had in store for them as a family. It was a race against time; the time that was the life of his little boy. He was prepared to break down all the barriers to carve his way through to a diagnosis, an achievement that would be against all odds. Now he and Sally are equally determined to turn their energies towards finding a treatment for their little son and all the other children in their extended HBSL family.

'We have something tangible to fight now that the disease has a name.'

Those lofty visions of the grand birthday parties that Sally had envisioned throwing when Massimo was growing inside her, like everything else in their lives, have been adapted to suit Massimo and ultimately make him happy. They don't take anything for granted these days.

'It's the small things that make us smile,' says Sally. 'It's such a delight for us that Massimo can go swimming once a week with his Uncle Johnny, who comes especially to his school, splashing around with him in the pool.'

Massimo loves playing with his brothers, both of whom are fiercely protective of him. Leonardo and Marco seem wise beyond their years. When Massimo's MRI results came back not long ago they announced to their kindergarten class that their brother was 'growing myelin'. The twins have even learned how to extract DNA from kiwi fruit. Often Sally will find the boys at home, seated on the couch with their toy laptops propped up in front of them, pretending to be Stephen emailing 'Dr Ryan'. Leonardo keeps a toy cup beside him, and picks it up from time to time, pretending to sip his 'espresso'. Marco takes breaks from their 'research' game to dance around to Taylor Swift songs, as they chat about how the team is making a special medicine to help their brother get better.

The twins are excited about Massimo's birthday coming up and aren't short of suggestions about what presents to buy. They've already chosen things they know their brother will love.

'They've been eyeing off a giant, brightly coloured squishy ball at our local toy store,' Sally says laughing. 'It will be a sensory delight for Massimo. Although he's engaging with the world more and more, there are still not many things he responds to in his communication book. "Birthday Party" is certainly one that grabs his attention, though, and it's a delight to see his face light up when we point to the icon of the birthday cake. I wonder if he even appreciates what a significant event it all really is.'

Sally pauses, and gazes across the room at Stephen

playing on the floor with Massimo. 'Given where we were only six years ago,' she says, 'each time we have the opportunity to celebrate another one of Massimo's birthdays, it truly is the greatest gift of all.'

ACKNOWLEDGEMENTS

Stephen and Sally Damiani:
We wouldn't be here penning these acknowledgements if it wasn't for the tireless efforts of Dr Leah Kaminsky, who has transformed our anecdotes, ramblings and sometimes vents into beautiful prose. Leah, we will be eternally grateful to you for believing in our story and dedicating so much of yourself over the past year to turning the laundry list of ideas we excitedly brainstormed around our dining table early in the new year into a book we are so immensely proud of.

We would also like to acknowledge the many other people who believed in our story and helped us share it beyond our small circle of family and friends. When we track back to how we got to this point, once again thank you, Leah, for your poignant, thought-provoking essay 'Promise or Peril, Revolution in our Genes'. Thank you, Julianne Schultz, Erica Sontheimer, Nick Bray and Susan Hornbeck, for sharing this essay with your readers in the

10th anniversary edition of the *Griffith REVIEW*. You kicked off the Massimo Effect, which saw our story shared with hundreds of thousands more people in the *Weekend Australian* and then a million more on ABC *Australian Story*. Thank you to Max Walker and the crew who put together our *Australian Story* – 'Cracking the Code'. We couldn't think of better people to have following us around with cameras. Your sensitivity and empathy made it easy for us to open up and share our story with all of your viewers. Finally, to Jacinta DiMase, Meredith Curnow and Sophie Ambrose for making this book a reality.

When we are constantly confronted with 'leuko-what?', the opportunity to share our story and create awareness about a condition as rare as Leukodystrophy is critically important, not just for us but for all the people touched by this insidious condition, be they the patients themselves or their family, friends and carers. Awareness is half the battle, so thank you all for contributing to the fight.

Ryan, we don't think we will ever feel we have thanked you enough for all that you have done. Thank you for taking on the challenge no one else wanted and for committing so much of yourself to getting the result you did. While we couldn't have solved the puzzle without everyone else bringing their pieces to the table, you put them all together. We cannot imagine ever getting to where we are today without you and will always be grateful, not just for what you have done but for what you continue to do.

We are forever grateful for the work of Rick Leventer, Adeline Vanderver, Marjo van der Knaap, Nicole Wolf and the army of clinicians and scientists behind the scenes who worked tirelessly to achieve the diagnosis. Our success was the results of many.

We would also like to acknowledge the many institutions that supported the attainment of Massimo's diagnosis and that continue to support the ongoing work of the Mission Massimo Foundation: University of Queensland – Institute for Molecular Bioscience, Brisbane, Australia; Royal Children's Hospital, Melbourne, Australia; Murdoch Children's Research Institute, Melbourne, Australia; Victorian Clinical Genetic Services, Melbourne, Australia; University of Queensland – Australian Institute for Bioengineering and Nanotechnology, Brisbane, Australia; University of New South Wales – Functional Genomics Group, Sydney, Australia; Walter and Eliza Hall Institute, Melbourne, Australia; Children's National Hospital, Washington DC, USA; VU University Medical Centre, Amsterdam.

We would like to acknowledge the generous support of Illumina. Thank you for believing in project 'Poor Little Dude' and continuing to unlock the genome. Thanks also for the invitation to participate in the Key Opinion Genomics Summit in San Diego in 2014.

We will always be grateful to the generous supporters of the Mission Massimo Foundation, including the many runners and volunteers at Run Melbourne 2014 and XCOR Space Expeditions. Your support has meant that this book has Chapters 12 and 13, and has – and will continue to – change the lives of people living with Leukodystrophy, as we turn science fiction into science fact. Watch this space for Chapter 14.

Even a book of this length covers only a small part of our story and does not do justice to the many amazing people in our lives. While not all of you appear in the pages of this book that is not to say you have not had an impact.

To our parents, Shane and Sally, brother, John, and uncle, Berge. We don't think that we can ever thank you enough for the endless hours of care and support. You have always been there when we have needed you, regardless of whether we have given you five days or five minutes notice. Without this support our lives would have fallen apart. Hilda, we know that if Alzheimer's disease hadn't taken you from us you would have been right by our side for this whole journey and probably would have had a go at finding the diagnosis yourself.

Thank you to all the friends – old and new – who showered us with support along the way; to the lads who were there to share a beer and tears during our darkest days, and the girls who rallied around and didn't let us endure this on our own. A special thank you to Nick Strong for his generous support of our research initiatives and seeing beyond rare disease to the broader long-term impact of this work on the prevention, diagnosis and treatment of many genetic diseases.

Brian Rabinowitz, thank you for being so much more than a trainer. You stopped Stephen from falling into the abyss and defied physics to get a front-row rugby union forward across the finish line of the Melbourne Marathon.

Jo, you once told us to stop thanking you, but you know we never will. You love Massimo as unconditionally as we do and we couldn't ask for more.

Siobhan, we only share a sliver of your involvement in our lives in the book, but thank you for sticking it out with us for so long and for being a 'super-nanny' when it came to getting all of the boys sleeping. Thank you also to Prue, the newest member of the 'care-crew'. You and Siobhan don't just care for our boys, but love them like your own.

Team Massimo grows outside of our home to include the many wonderful and most often completely selfless carers, therapists, teachers and doctors who all play their part in taking care of Massimo. Thank you to all of the clinicians and therapists at the Royal Children's Hospital for your ongoing care of Massimo and for coming along on this journey into the unknown with us.

When Massimo is not at home we cannot think of a better place for him to be than the amazing Glenallen School. Our heartfelt thanks to all of the educators, therapists and carers there who support Massimo to reach his full potential each and every day.

To the brave children and their families around the world fighting HBSL and other Leukodystrophies, your strength and courage inspire us to move medical science forward and develop treatments every single day. We stay together, we survive.

Massimo, thank you for being such a fighter each and every day, for never giving up and for giving the world's best hugs. You might not realise it just now but you have had more impact on medical science than any little boy we've known. We love you to Mars and back.

Marco and Leonardo, you have brought Mum, Dad and Massimo so much joy. One day when you are older you may read this book and it will help you to understand how incredibly special you both are to us.. In your few short years you have taught us so much, most importantly what it means to be a family. You may not have come to us in the most conventional way, but we wouldn't have it any other way. Melinda, we think about you each and every day. Thank you for helping us grow our family from the ashes of 24 July 2009.

To Stephen for being one of the most determined people on the planet and for not being afraid to push the envelope when it all seemed impossible.

Leah Kaminsky:
In addition to everyone Sally and Stephen have already thanked, I would like to acknowledge Glenfern Studios, the Victorian Writers' Centre and Varuna the Writers' House for space and time to work on this book. I have felt so privileged to be part of the Damiani family's life. Telling their story has helped me appreciate the love of my own family even more than I already did. Yohanan, Alon, Ella and Maia Loeffler are my constant inspiration and support. Brendan Higgins and Daryl Karp always have my back. So many, many others have held my writer's hand, and even though our DNA would tell otherwise, Sandra Levin is my dearest sister.